SECRETS
OF
HEALING BACK PAIN

By Dr. Craig Zion Cain, D.C.

ISBN: 1439225303
ISBN-13: 9781439225301

SECRETS OF HEALING BACK PAIN

Finally, a self help book that teaches you
how to care for your own back!

By Dr. Craig Zion Cain, D.C.

TABLE OF CONTENTS

....

INTRODUCTION

....

You are already perfect. It's not something we have to get; it's something we have to remember!

If you understand and follow this book, I believe you can begin to heal and keep your back in great shape. This book is written due to my own struggle with back pain. It took many years to pick through the mire to find out not only the causes of most back pain but also the steps towards its cure. This book is not written to replace your chiropractor or treatments from you favorite health care practitioner, It is written to allow you to do your part in maintaining your own back.

Once your back is in shape you should still see your chiropractor. Life is adjusting us whether we know it or not. If you have a re-injury you may have to see your chiropractor a bit more than you want, but as soon as you can, you can start to stabilize your back at home and hold your alignments so that you will feel better between chiropractic visits.

There are many related factors involved with this process of getting your back to feel better: your lifestyle, stress level, exercise program, and diet, just to name a few. Understanding these ten chapters, essentially, are steps to a better life without back pain. But first you will need to know what's causing your back pain, which is step one. To understand this, you have to know a little bit of anatomy. So here it goes. Let's start with anatomy; once you get through this, the rest is easy!

DEDICATION

....

I dedicate this book to my lovely wife Eika for her love, wisdom and unfailing support. I also dedicate this book to my two children, Sho and Zia for their love and companionship!

MEDICAL/HEALTH DISCLAIMER

....

The information provided in this book should not be construed as personal medical advice or instruction. No action should be taken based solely on the contents of this book.

Readers should consult appropriate health professionals on any matter relating to their health and well being, they should consult appropriate health professionals on any matter relating to the health.

The information and opinions provided here are believed to be accurate and sound, based on the best judgment available to the author, but readers who fail to consult appropriate health authorities assume the risk of any injuries. This author is not responsible for errors or omissions.

QUICK START GUIDE

....

Many individuals who are interested in this book may not necessarily be interested in reading, in detail, all the information presented in the first two chapters. Some of you reading this book may want to know just the essentials and start right into some of the other sections of this book. Strong areas of interest may be chapter 3 on what to do when your back hurts and chapters 5 and 6, the exercise and stretching portions of this book. Of course I encourage you to read all areas of this book, but I realize that we all have different interests and for this reason I've put the essentials or the minimum you need to know before delving into these other chapters of this book, into a quick start guide. These "essentials" I feel you need to know are underlined in the first two chapters. The first two chapters do have quite a bit of anatomy and physiology and many of you folks do want to know, in detail, all about how your back functions. For those, please read everything. But for those who don't care to know all that information, follow the quick start areas of chapters one and two and then get into the rest of the book. The main thing is to start to heal your own back pain today and enjoy the process!

CHAPTER ONE

....

What you need to know
A crash course in back anatomy

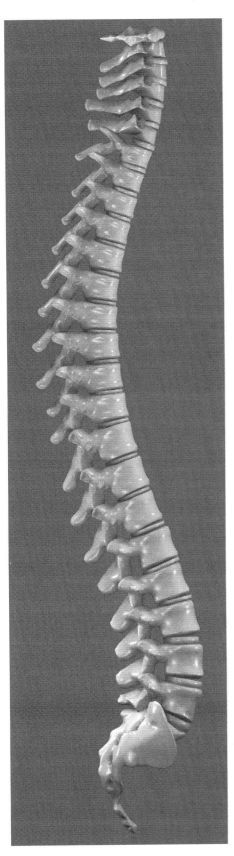

The spine is made up of 7 cervical vertebrae, 12 thoracic vertebrae, and 5 lumbar vertebrae. At the base of the spine is your sacrum. The sacrum is made up of 5 fused bones together. At the bottom of the sacrum is your tailbone. So there are four distinct areas of your spine. Each of the four areas of the spine has a curve. The cervical has a lordodic curve that curves in; the thoracic has a kyphotic curve that curves out; the lumbar has a lordodic curve that curves in again; and the sacrum a kyphotic curve, curving out again. These curves act as springs to guard us against the forces of gravity. When an individual does not have a proper curve in one of these areas, this area can become injured. Each vertebra in the spine is attached to the vertebra above and the vertebra below. Between each vertebra is a disc. This disc is firmly attached to the bone of the vertebra above and the vertebra below. The vertebrae articulate with each other; or, in other words, the vertebrae have a joint linking one vertebra with another. All of these joints from the base of the spine at the sacrum to the top of the spine just below the skull have a saggital (or, in layman's terms, a straight surface) that lets the vertebra above rest up against the vertebra below. Then that vertebra butts up to the following one below it, and so on. Each vertebra is cradled, if you will, from the vertebra above and the vertebra below. When vertebrae are in place where they should be, their discs are also in a good and normal position, which allows the nerve roots that exit under each vertebra to transfer the nerve fluid from the spine into the surrounding musculature and into the rest of the body.

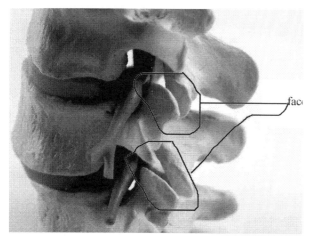

If you can get a good picture of all this, then you can begin to understand how back pain arises and more importantly how back pain can be alleviated. When one of these vertebrae are slightly out of place it causes problems.

Subluxation

When the vertebra is slightly out of place, it is called a subluxation. A subluxation is a misaligned vertebra. The funny thing is, in most all cases, the vertebrae misalign in the same direction. If you look at the human spine from the side, you will see all the vertebrae and how each area of the spine has a curve (recall the four curves of the spine discussed briefly above). The front of the body is called the anterior portion, and the rear (or back) of the spine is called the posterior portion. The way the spine is made from near the top of the spine at the 2nd cervical all the way down to the sacrum, all the vertebrae misalign in a posterior direction. Because the spine almost always subluxates or misaligns in a posterior direction (in other words, the vertebra moves backwards to subluxate), the vertebra can often be realigned by pushing from the back towards the front.

The spine was designed perfectly to be manipulated with the hands. If the vertebrae did not have these saggital facets intercepting the vertebra, chiropractors or osteopaths would not have a chance in the world to bring about proper alignment with an adjustment.

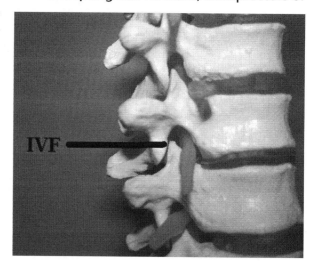

Let's review. We have 7 cervical vertebrae in the neck, 12 thoracic vertebrae in the upper and mid back (ribs are connected to them), 5 big lumbar vertebrae, and at the bottom, below the lumbar spine, we have the sacrum. Between each of these 25 vertebrae, there are discs. Exiting out from under each vertebra is a spinal nerve one on the left, one on the right. You can see from the drawing below that there is a space right next to the facet joint and the disc. It is an orifice or hole called the intervertebral foramen or IVF. The point is, when the vertebra misaligns and moves into a backward or posterior position, this hole becomes smaller and it also causes swelling in this area putting pressure on the nerve exiting through this hole.

NORMAL   SUBLUXATION

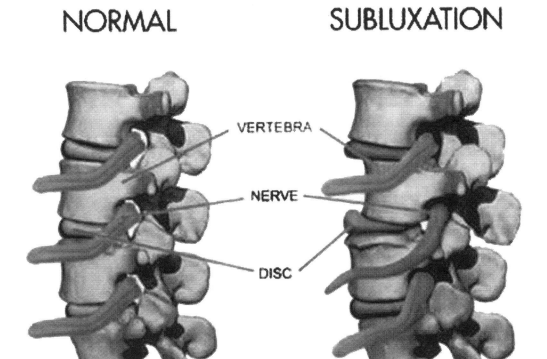

VERTEBRA

NERVE

DISC

Now look at the drawing; housed in the posterior part of the spine is the spinal cord. If the vertebra moves or misaligns, it not only makes the IVF smaller but causes the disc to move closer to the spinal column. There is a sac covering the spinal cord called the thecal sac. Within the thecal sac is the cerebral spinal fluid, or CSF. The thecal sac is extremely sensitive, and when touched upon by the disc during subluxation, it can cause extreme pain; This pain can often times feel "electric".

"In a nutshell..."

Basically, the curves in your spine are there for a reason. It is normal anatomy that needs to be maintained. If you decrease or reverse your curves by flexing forward (like slouching in a chair), you can subluxate your back. All 24 bones in your back (except the very top vertebra, called the Atlas) are able to move posterior, or backwards when the vertebrae subluxate. In other words, the vertebrae move from front to the back of your body when they misalign. By flexing forward, you can move the vertebrae out of place. Does this mean you should never flex forward? No.
When doing Yoga, for example, some postures flex the spine forward. If your spine is in good shape, it will add to your flexibility. If working out in the gym with weights and you do an exercise that flexes you forward, it is a bad idea, unless you have no back pain (being in the vicinity of 18 years old would be a plus, too!). Always use caution when flexing the spine forward.

Most of the time, low back pain is caused from slouching in a chair or car. Improper lifting; Example, by flexing the spine and not using your legs to do the work is another major cause of injury.

Remember, the spine and its 25 moveable vertebra cannot, by design, move anterior or forward, although they can move backward and get caught in a misaligned position. By not flexing forward, especially while lifting anything heavy, you will most definitely avoid many an injury.

CHAPTER TWO

....

What causes back pain?
What causes subluxation or misalignment?

Usually what causes subluxation of one of the vertebrae to move into a posterior position is flexion of the spine. What is flexion? Flexion of the spine occurs when the spine bends toward the front of the body, like when standing and touching your toes. Doing things like bending over and picking up something or slouching in a chair causes the spine to flex. Also sleeping in a bed that is too soft can cause the spine to flex during sleep.

I recommend before doing anything in this book, that you check with your favorite doctor to make sure that you do not have any physical abnormalities in your spine. Some folks have congenital problems (something you were born with) that cause them back problems. These problems are best seen with an xray or an MRI. The X-ray photographs the bony structures, while the MRI, the soft tissues, discs and nerves. Also I recommend before doing any of the exercises in this book that you have a physical from your M.D. to make sure you are free of any underlying medical conditions that may arise while doing the exercises, stretching or aerobic exercises mentioned in this book.

Degeneration

Degeneration can be seen both with X-ray and MRI. Degeneration takes time to occur, so usually it is seen in people 30 or 40 years of age or older. If degeneration is present, it means there has been a long-standing problem for many years.

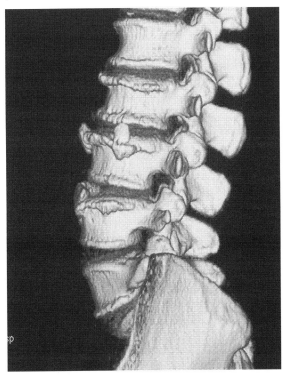

What causes degeneration? Basically subluxation causes degeneration. A misaligned vertebra or a subluxated vertebra is not in a normal position. Because of this abnormal position, the bone does not move normally during motion. That is why when I examine a patient, I always check the motion of the vertebra. Subluxated vertebrae always exhibit from a slight lack of motion to absolutely no motion at all. Can we feel this lack of motion? Yes, absolutely. As chiropractors, we are trained to feel motion of the vertebrae. All Kiso Practitioners are also trained in motion palpation of the spine.

The Cainzian Factor

I have postulated this theory due to the fact that no one else in medical research has coined a phrase for this daily occurrence in our bodies. Have you ever felt a spasm in your back muscles? Undoubtedly, since that it's one of the aches and pains of being human. It is difficult to go through life without ever having a back spasm. OK, so we have back spasms. When you get one, do they disappear right away? Sometimes they do and sometimes they don't. If you have had a back spasm that is re-occurring or one that doesn't seem to go away, have you tried rubbing it away? Or have you gone to a massage therapist? Well, what was the result? If you are experiencing muscle spasm due to the Cainzian factor, usually the muscle spasm does not go away at all or for very long. For example: You suddenly get a muscle spasm in your back, touch the area of pain, and – ouch! – you determine that's just what it is. Day after day, this spasm is still hanging around, and you surmise: "Oh, well, I'm just getting older! I guess I can't do that anymore." You set up a massage therapy session, but afterwards, it not only didn't go away, but now it is worse.

"What is going on? What is causing this?" you ask yourself.

This is actually a common occurrence. What is causing this is the Cainzian Factor. Let me explain further. When a subluxation occurs, because the bone moves posterior or towards the back of the body, it also brings the disc, which is firmly attached to the vertebra, also into a posterior position. There are two structures that the disc runs into on its way into this posterior position. One is the spinal nerve root (remember you have these nerve roots exiting the spine through the hole, or the IVF). The second structure is the spinal cord itself. As the vertebra subluxates, it brings the disc closer to these two structures.

What is in the nerve fluid that flows from the spine into the nerve roots and into the musculature of the body? Axonal fluid. This fluid gives muscles oxygen and nutrients. In addition to this, information also flows back up these nerves, through the nerve roots and up the spine to be received by the brain.

The point that I am making is this: <u>When muscle does not get enough nerve fluid from the nerve in question, the muscle spasms! It is a defense mechanism of the body. As you know, we have many defense mechanisms in our finely tuned bodies. When the muscle senses a lack of fluid from the nerve, the muscle spasms to protect the injured area. Why isn't there enough fluid? Because of the subluxation cutting off or limiting the flow of nerve fluid from the spine.</u>

As the vertebra moves backward towards the spinal cord and nerve roots, the area swells. All of these actions compromise the fluid flow coming from the nerve root. This is the Cainzian Factor. It is real and it is affecting us everyday of our lives. <u>So, instead of massaging the muscle over and over again, fix the subluxation and the muscle will calm down all on its own.</u> Now if you were to get a massage after this had been alleviated, it would really feel good and you would reap the benefits so much more.

Symptoms

Let's start from the top down. Symptoms vary greatly with subluxation. It depends where the subluxated vertebra is. If it is in the upper neck, it can cause headaches and radiating pain from the back of the head over the top of the scalp to the inside of the eyes. It can also affect your ears. Usually this particular subluxation is caused from the Atlas vertebra or the occiput being misaligned. The Atlas Vertebra is at the top of the spine next to the scull. This vertebra is the one exception, instead of moving posterior it travels from side to side, subluxating left or right.

Now the problem is not that simple. When the vertebra subluxates left, it often causes the cranium (your head) to subluxate right. So your pain from having this problem can be felt on the left or right or both. So far we have not talked about the cranium. The back part of the skull called the occiput (part of the cranium), connects with the atlas vertebra. The subluxated atlas and cranium cause pain and muscle spasm, which, in turn, cause radiation of pain to the back of the head and into one or both ears. It can also radiate pain into the jaw. When this area is subluxated it can create a radiating pain that goes from the back of the head, over the top of the skull and into the inside of the eyebrows. This is a classic trigger point pattern, or referred pain pattern. It can also affect the eustachian tube. This tube drains the middle ear and is responsible for the popping sound you experience when going from a high altitude to a lower altitude. This tube runs from the middle ear into the nasal area. It gets blocked sometimes when you have a cold and can also become blocked from the upper cervical area in your neck being out of alignment and causing muscle spasm in this area. This can contribute to frequent ear infections.

What are trigger points?

Trigger points are bunched up muscles. They were named and discovered by Janet Travell, M.D. Trigger points are described as hyper-irritable spots usually in a taut band of skeletal muscle, or its fascia, that is painful on compression and can give rise to characteristic referred pain. Trigger point therapy has been around awhile and is used all over the world. But I believe that the origin of why trigger points manifest is in many cases due to a hyper irritable nerve/muscular situation called the Cainzian factor.

The origin of a "trigger point" or, for lack of a better word, a muscle spasm, is in many cases caused by the Cainzian Factor. The compromised nerve flow of a nerve has caused a lack of fluid to reach the muscle in question. <u>This muscle has spasmed due to its innate defense mechanism, which is to protect the body from further harm.</u>

When a muscle senses a decrease in axonal nerve flow, it is designed to spasm. The spasm will usually "flow" in a line either from the sciatic nerve plexus in the lower spine or from the brachial nerve plexus in the lower neck. The brachial nerve plexus flows from the 5th cervical vertebra to the 1st thoracic vertebra. The 5 nerve roots become three trunks that branch down the arms. So if you have numbness or tingling in the fingers, it may mean the nerve root in the brachial plexus has been compromised by subluxation.

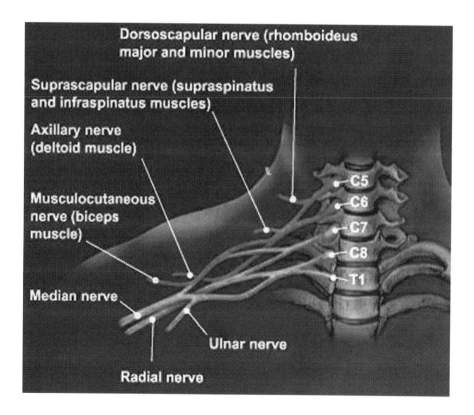

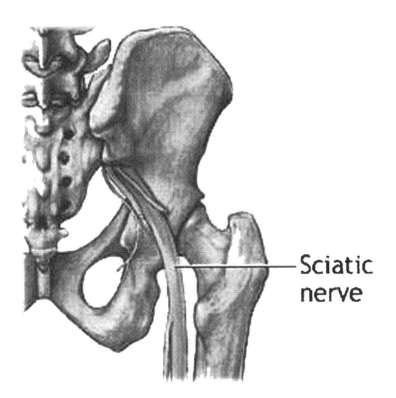

Sciatic
nerve

Let me explain this in greater detail. The sciatic nerve plexus located in the lumbar area is made up of 5 nerve roots. The sciatic nerve originates from the 1 lumbar down to the sacrum. It is the largest nerve in the body, flowing from the low back into the buttocks and down the legs into the feet. So if you have pain in your calf, it may be due to a subluxated vertebra affecting the sciatic nerve. If you have a muscle spasm in the right buttocks you may find another spasm in the back of the leg and another in the calf, following the sciatic nerve down the leg. If you find a muscle spasm or trigger point in the right side of the neck, you may find another trigger point in the right shoulder, another in the back of the right upper arm, and so on, following the brachial nerve down the right arm. These muscle spasms found running in a line originate from the nerve feeding that muscle. When the muscle senses a decrease in nerve flow, the muscle spasms in various place along the nerve path.

Here are just some of the symptoms caused by subluxation:
Seeing a list like this can conjure up a negative feeling, but I would like to list these symptoms to let you know the different ways that subluxation can manifest.

List of symptoms caused by subluxation

HEAD AREA
* Jaw pain
* Radiating pain around the ear
* Full feeling in the ear or ears
* Pain radiating from the back of the skull into the scalp
  and moving towards the inside of the eyes
* Pain in the front of the neck
* Unable to turn the neck due to pain
* Sharp hot feeling, pain from the back of the neck, either
  moving up the skull or down the neck
* Tingling in the face
* Hair on the scalp tingling

LOWER NECK AND SHOULDER AREA
* Pain on top of the shoulders
* Unable to turn the neck due to muscle spasm
* Pain in the shoulder
* Pain in the arm
* Cramping or a clamping feeling in the upper or lower arm
* Pain in the wrist and hand
* Numbness in the arm or fingers, usually one, two, or three fingers
* Weakness of the arm, hand and fingers
* Hair standing up somewhere on the arm
* Head bent to one side, unable to correct the position

THORACIC REGION FROM UPPER BACK THROUGH THE MID BACK
* Sharp pain in the shoulder blade area
* Sharp pain around the spine
* Sharp pain that hurts more when you take a deep breath
* Sharp pain that radiates from the back into the front of the chest
* Dull soreness in the kidney area

LOWER BACK AREA
* Dull soreness around the waist or higher
* Pain on one side of the lower back radiating to the kidney area
* Pain in the buttock at one point
* Pain radiating into the groin and front of the thighs
* Pain in the knees

* Pain in the calf muscles
* Pain at the heel or heels
* Burning into the buttock
* Burning in the back of the leg
* Burning into the groin
* Burning in the calf, especially the outside of the calf
* Burning in the heal and foot
* Numbness or weakness anywhere in the leg or foot
* Hair standing on end anywhere on the leg
* Numbness in the big toe or toes

Does massage help muscle spasm?

Yes, it usually does; however, muscle spasm often times is caused by a hyper irritable nerve situation. So if you find that massage only temporarily makes the muscle spasm better and the muscle spasm returns quickly after massaging it, it is a good indication that it is caused by the Cainzian Factor. For a muscle spasm to occur and manifest without the Cainzian Factor, the muscle has to be over strained (using it too much).

Other factors that may cause muscle spasms are dehydration or lack of magnesium and calcium. Basically, if the electrolyte balance is off in your body, this can trigger widespread muscle spasms. I'm sure all of you reading this book have experienced muscle spasms that were only temporarily relieved by massage. You pay for a good massage and two hours later the pain returns. The Cainzian Factor is the culprit. How do we fix muscle spasms caused by the Cainzian Factor? By adjusting the spine! That's right, relieving subluxation. Does a chiropractor have to be involved in the adjusting process to relieve subluxation? Not always.....this is the SECRET of relieving back pain!

Other symptomatology can be rather interesting. Did you know that spinal subluxation can cause symptoms like anxiety, frightful feelings, etc. It is true. There are two parts to your nervous system: a YIN and a YANG function. The Yin part is known as the parasympathetic nervous system. It allows you to rest, restore, and rejuvenate. It lowers your blood pressure; it lowers your heart rate, and makes you feel sleepier sometimes. The other part, or Yang part, is known as your sympathetic nervous system. The sympathetic nervous system makes you tense. It increases both your blood pressure and heart rate, and makes it difficult to take a deep breath. If left "out of alignment" for a while, it can manifest into panic attacks and anxiety.

The sympathetic nervous system can cause "stress" hormones to be released into your body. One set of these hormones are called catecholamines. They circulate in your body like little "pac-men", eating away at your tissues. It functions as one of the human body's defense mechanisms. This sympathetic nervous system is also known as your "fight or flight" mechanism. Fight or flight means that when threatened by an external danger (such as a bear coming at you), it will circulate catecholamines in order to liberate energy from your tissues to "boost" your energy level temporarily, so you can run faster (who wants to fight a bear anyway?).

But the problem is this: This defense mechanism is only supposed to last a short time. As I said at the introduction of this book, we have bodies designed 160,000 years ago, but now that we live in the digital age, we sometimes have prolonged stress that our bodies and minds have never dealt with before. When the sympathetic nervous system is out of balance with the para-sympathetic nervous system, it is called a sympathetic override. In other words the sympathetic nervous system is "overriding" the parasympathetic nervous system. It is supposed to function interchangeably as you live your daily life. Yet when we have a sympathetic override, you won't have that balance between the two systems. You become so tired from your sympathetic nervous system being "ON" too long that you become overwhelmed, resulting in sleeplessness and high levels of stress.

So how does this occur? Three things cause this sympathetic override. One is having too much stress in your life. Two is having a subluxation in the spine because the sympathetic and the parasympathetic nervous systems have actual physical areas in the spine. Look at any anatomy book, and you'll find it. The para-sympathetic nervous system is located in two areas. It is located in the upper most part of your neck down to the 5th cervical vertebra in your neck. It is also located in your sacrum, the sacred bone. The sympathetic nervous system is physically located between the neck and sacrum, mostly in the thoracic spinal region. If you have a subluxation in the upper neck, for instance, it can shut off the parasympathetic nervous system like "a light switch." Conversely, if you have a subluxation in the thoracic region, you can have a para-sympathetic override. This will make you feel extremely heavy and lethargic. Isn't this fascinating! Now for the third reason: The sympathetic override can also be caused by pressure on your dura mater.

What is the dura mater?

Dura mater

The dura mater is the covering you have over your brain and spinal cord. It allows the cerebral spinal fluid (CSF) to circulate. There is a healing method called Sacral-occipital technique or SOT. This healing technique was created by a chiropractor named Dr. DeJarnette. He surmised that manipulating the cranial bones could influence your health, both mental and physical. Also earlier in history, Dr. John E. Upledger, an American Osteopathic surgeon, expounded on a concept developed by another osteopathic doctor William G. Sutherland in the 1930's. Upledger named this technique Cranial-Sacral therapy. These wonderful methods are practiced all over the world. These two methods use light pressure exerted on the cranial bones and sacrum to "open up" the flow of CSF. When the CSF flow is normalized, it causes-- or rather, *allows* greater health!

The whole point of these techniques function around a rhythm that exists and that can be felt in the cranial bones and in the body itself. This rhythm is caused by the body's circulation of this Cerebral Spinal Fluid, which circulates around the brain and through the spinal cord by means of three "pumps". The Sacral-occipital technique and Cranial-sacral therapy primarily treat two of the pumps. Both techniques treat the cranial bones and the sacrum. The cranial bones "flare" out to cause a pumping action, forcing CSF down the spine, but the sacrum at the bottom of the spine also has a "pumping" action (the third pump), which circulates the CSF back up the spine to the brain. The occiput is the second part of the cranial-sacral pump system. It is located in the back of the skull where the cranium and first cervical vertebrae meet. The dura mater is connected all the way around the foremen magnum at this meeting and the dura mater is also connected partially at the 2nd and 3rd cervical vertebrae a as well as to the 2nd sacral tubercle. The Dura mater is extremely sensitive in these areas because these are the only places the dura mater is actually connected to anything in the spine (it is mostly free floating). When the pumping mechanisms don't function correctly, the CSF does not function normally. When this occurs, it can cause learning disabilities and all kinds of abnormal feelings. Another thing that it causes is an abnormality in the sympathetic/parasympathetic nervous system. What happens is this: When you have a subluxation at the primary site which is either the occiput or the 1st cervical vertebra (the atlas), or even a subluxation at the 2nd or 3rd cervical vertebrae, these misalignments can cause a malfunction of the cranial-sacral system. This malfunction to the second part of the cranial-sacral system is caused by "pressure" on the dura mater located in the area of subluxation. This pressure on the dura mater is seen as a threat by our bodies. Again, it is another defense mechanism we have. Pressure on the dura mater causes a fight or flight response to occur. Because the dura mater is connected all the way around the foremen magnum, it is likely to me that this area may influence the flow of CSF even more than the first part of the cranial-sacral system, the cranial bones.

There has been a lot of controversy with the Sacral-occipital technique and craniosacral therapy and the theory of manipulating the cranial bones. This controversy exists mostly because the cranial bones are connected together by very strong sutures that do not allow much movement to occur. So applying these techniques to "influence" CSF flow is to some degree doubtful in many people's eyes. I do on the other hand believe in what they do and have experienced it firsthand. I always enjoy the treatments and feel "better" afterwards. Yet if the Sacral-occipital technique and craniosacral therapy don't treat this second "pump," then what can be done about it? Over 20 years and more than 50, 000 treatments later, I have developed the Kiso Method. It manipulates not only the second part of the cranio-sacral pump, but the sacrum as well. However, this method will not be discussed in this book. If you feel you have a serious problem with the sympathetic/para-sympathetic nervous system, you should go to a Kiso practitioner to have this "fixed". Kiso practitioners are not only chiropractors but also massage therapists, acupuncturists, as well as sacro-occipital therapists, cranio-sacral therapists and rolfers. But there are things you can do at home (and not do at home for that matter) that can make you feel much better. These "things" cannot only help back pain and headaches, but also help with anxiety and other associated problems.

Now, if you've made it this far without being too confused, the rest is easy!

CHAPTER THREE

....

What To Do When Your Back Hurts

You know a bit about anatomy and the spine now. Actually, you may know more about how back pain occurs than many doctors. The reason for this fact is because most medical doctors have no idea how a chiropractor is going to help a person with a subluxated and painful back. They are not taught this in medical school and focus their attention on "allopathic" medicine. You also understand a little about how we are influenced by subluxation and how it can affect our lives. Back pain can influence our emotions and limit our movements and strength as well as cause irritation and debilitating pain.

Knowing how subluxation occurs, it is easy to understand how spinal pain and associated muscle spasm can often be alleviated when the subluxated vertebra is pushed "IN". Remember, most muscle spasm in the spine and their radiating pain are caused by subluxation.

So how exactly can the displaced vertebrae be pushed back into the spine from posterior to anterior (or from back of the body to the front)? First, there needs to be some means of accomplishing this, and I have just the thing! A ball. It is about 6 inches or 16 cm in diameter. I call it the Kiso Ball; it is small enough to lie on and tough enough to withstand the weight of 300 pounds of pressure, but soft enough not to irritate the spine. Using hard objects to accomplish this task can injure the spine and ribs. The Kiso Ball can be used from the low back and sacral area up to the upper neck.

Using the Kiso Ball

Let's start with laying face up on carpet, if possible (if you have a hardwood floor, it is fine too, just a little harder on the body). Now, put your knees up, bringing your heels

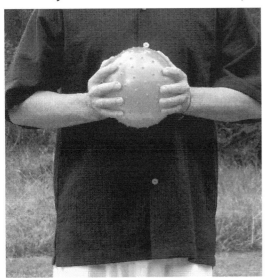

five or six inches from your buttocks. Raise your hips up high and put the Kiso Ball into the small of your lower back (refer to the picture). Now, rest with the ball under your low back, making sure your pelvis is extending over the ball while stabilizing the ball under you by putting your arms out to the side and resting them on the floor. Now with your knees up, open your legs.

Note: If you hear a "pop" in your back, that is fine. Don't worry about the sound; the "popping" sound you often hear in your back when you move (or when being adjusted by your chiropractor) is just gas. All the joints in the spine are "air tight", so when they expand enough, they let in gas. A gas exchange causes a noise, kind of like putting your palms together and rapidly pulling them apart. This movement causes a suction noise. Try it with your own hands. See, it's nothing to worry about. Many people think the bone is cracking when they hear this noise, but no harm is being done. Actually this lets your joints in your back expand. Lying face up with the ball under your low back while letting your knees open up usually feels good.

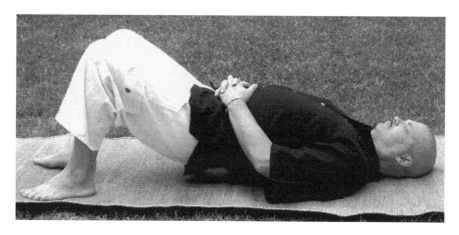

Just lie there in this position for about 15 seconds. Now, you can move the ball up a bit higher towards your mid back. You do this by lifting up your pelvis from the ball, tucking in your heels and stabilizing with your arms on the floor at both sides, as you "crab walk" to reposition the Kiso Ball, sliding it from the low back up to the mid back. Once in the desired position, lie on your side and pull the ball out. You are done with the low back.

The Kiso Ball for your neck to mid back Lying on your back still, same position as before with your arms out to the side for stability and your knees up and heels near your buttocks, but the ball under your upper back.

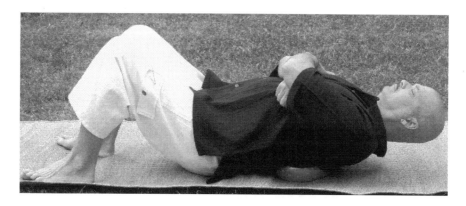

Let your neck extend over the ball at the spot where the "knob" or "hump" of the upper back meets the neck. It should be comfortable and relaxing. It may be a little sore if you have a problem in this area (note, if you have extreme soreness, see your chiropractor or Kiso practitioner as soon as possible). Now with the crab-like motion, slide your body up over the ball, allowing it to travel down your spine from the upper back to the mid back. Remember you have already done your low back so you only need to go about mid way down your back, but if you like and it is comfortable, you can let the ball go all the way down to the low back again.

* A warning: Do not flex the spine while performing this procedure.

Flexing the spine means to "curl" the spine forward. Remember, flexing the spine is how most spinal injuries occur. You can "flex" the spine in two ways doing this procedure: One is putting the ball under the head, which flexes the neck forward, and the other way is to put the ball under the tail bone area, which again flexes the low back forward. Avoid doing these two things.

I recommend using the Kiso Ball 1 to 4 times per week, depending on your back pain level. Numerous patients in my clinic have used this procedure for years. I know it works; the results are actually incredible. You might think this is a "practice management" mistake. But I believe, the more you can help patients, even if it is doing it themselves at home, the more referrals I will receive in my practice. We never have a "lack" of patients at my clinic so I believe it to be true. I've had patients tell me enthusiastically "your cutting your own throat, teaching me the ball thing." I love it. I'm not "cutting my own throat." I'm helping them – and that's what I'm supposed to do! It is such a simple procedure. It takes literally two minutes to perform, but it can make a massive difference in your level of back pain. On occasions when you have a severe onset of low back pain. See your chiropractor or Kiso practitioner before using the Kiso ball. On these occasions, when you have severe pain, this will mean you probably have disc swelling and the Kiso ball will not be enough. Just a cautionary note.

What are some other things you can do?

You can use a smaller, harder ball, called the Chibi Ball. This is for muscle spasms rather than for relieving subluxation. It is great for putting pressure on muscle spasms that are found in the upper back (the trapezius muscles or in muscles around the scapula). It can also be used near the back of the armpit, because these muscles often have muscle spasms. You can also try laying slightly on your side and plant the chibi ball in the middle of your gluteal muscles, this feels great!

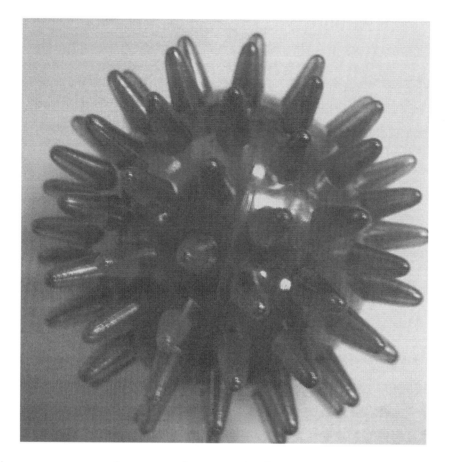

The other area you may have muscle spasm is along the sides of the spine (not on the spine because there are no muscles located there). Right down the center of the spine you have bumps called the spinous processes that come from the vertebrae. Many times these spinous processes are irregular in shape; so you may become alarmed if you feel that one is bigger than another. Many patients start to wonder what's this or that in their spine. They will ask me, "Look at this bump; I've never seen it before. Is it normal?" Don't worry. This often happens when one starts to "pay attention" to their spine for the first time. After a while these "new" findings will dissipate.

To relieve muscle pain in the plantar of the foot, sit in a chair and put your foot on the Chibi Ball, using it to massage the area of pain. Another use for the Chibi Ball is in the gluteus (or butt) muscles, which often get spasms.

Kiso meditation cushion treatments

This is good for the entire spine. The Kiso meditation cushions are very firm and supportive. There are three main areas in the spine that can benefit from their use.

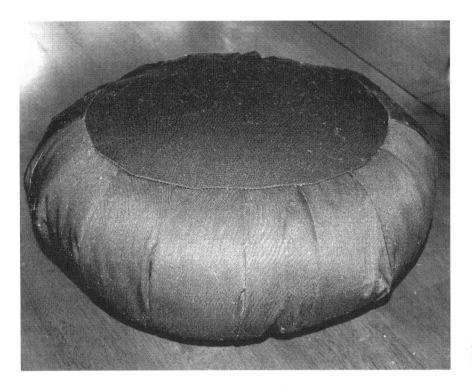

1) Cervical stretch

To perform this wonderful stretch and therapeutic maneuver, you put the cushion under the upper back and, with your knees bent and your toes pushing and lifting your knee up off the floor, you can position yourself raising your buttocks, making your back horizontal with the floor. Now you can extend the neck over the cushion and breathe in this position three long breaths.

2) Thoracic extension

To perform this anti-aging maneuver, you will be in the same position as the cervical stretch, except the cushion will be under your rib cage in the middle of your thoracic area. Now allow your shoulders, arms and upper back to extend over the cushion for three long breaths.

3) Lumbar extension

In this maneuver, you will position the cushion under your lumbar spine. Put your heels close to your buttocks and allow your knees to fall, one on the right and one on the left, while your upper back is resting on the floor. Take three long breaths in this extended position.

All the maneuvers using the Kiso cushion feel great and are beneficial for anti-aging. As we grow older, we tend to curl in on ourselves. What I mean is that our chest and shoulders curl in and the upper back becomes rounder, creating a larger kyphotic curve. This is due in part to our muscles and tendons becoming shorter and tighter in the front of the body, and our back muscles becoming weaker. We need to reverse this process by doing extension maneuvers and by strengthening the back.

Other back treatments

THE KISO CERVICAL LIFT

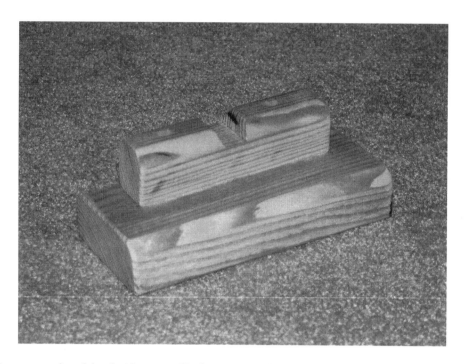

This is a wooden block, if you will, that is used to put pressure at the junction of your cranium and your atlas at the point of the foramen magnum. Remember, it's this area that is not only part of the cranio-sacral system, but also an area, when touched, makes the para-sympathetic nervous system activated. This wooden block is put under your neck while laying face up in the corpse pose. Once the block is in place, you may do abdominal breathing for one to three minutes. This treatment not only stimulates the para-sympathetic nervous system, but also stretches the neck, creating a desirable extension in the neck. It can also release the cervical area "pushing" the vertebrae forward. This maneuver is great for those individuals who have what is termed a reversed curve in the neck, or a "straight" cervical spine. Remember the cervical spine naturally has a 35 degree lordodic curve. If you have a reversed curve, this means your lordodic curve is basically gone. It's now straight or slightly reversed.

Aligning the hips

A good way to naturally align the hips is to lay face up and bring both your knees up. With both knees up, push on the outside of the knees towards the center using your palms. As you push, resist the pressure exerted by your arms by pushing out with your knees. With isometric pressure (staying in the same position), push and resist for about 10 seconds, do this up to three times. Now with both knees up again, push down with your palm on the right knee, resisting with isometric pressure while pulling at the same time, your left knee with your left hand. Do this simultaneously with isometric pressure for 10 seconds and do this up to three times. Now switch knees. Pulling up with the right knee and pushing down with the left using isometric pressure. This can often align the hips without worrying which hip is higher or which hip is lower. In many cases it self adjusts the hips naturally.

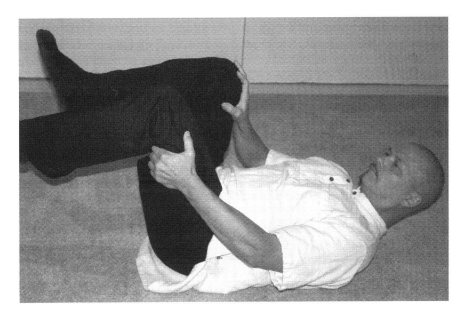

The shower Kiso position

Actually it was several of my patients who came up with this one. When I do my non-force Kiso Method on my patient's low back, I have them go on their knees on my Kiso Bench, which helps support their chest and I have my patients basically on all fours sticking their butt out and dropping their stomachs to create a lordodic curve. Once they have increased their lordotic curve to their maximum, I push down on the subluxated vertebra and do my Kiso oscillations to put the vertebra back into position without pain. Well, a few of my patients told me that when in severe low back pain, they get into the "Kiso Position" and stay there for a few minutes to make themselves feel better. I have a variation on this theme, get into the Kiso position while in the shower. One day, when I hurt my low back lifting a TV and slipping at the same time, I started to get fairly severe low back pain. I tried the Kiso Ball, it helped but I was still in pain. So when I took my evening shower, I assumed the "Kiso Position", basically on all fours, increasing my lordodic curve to the maximum, allowing my stomach to drop as much as possible, and letting the very hot water beat on my low back for about 3 minutes. WOW~ It helped a lot! I was about 40 percent better after my shower. So now, when my low back hurts, I assume the position in the shower to help ease muscle spasm associated with pain. To safely do this, you should be at a pain level of no greater than a 5.

Hot and cold packs

Hot and Cold packs are another fantastic way to relieve an aching back. When should ice be used? As a rule, use a genuine ice pack (including the gel "ice" packs). In other words, don't use frozen peas (for example) to put on your back.

USING ICE

I do not recommend using an ice pack on the upper and mid neck. You can use ice on your lower neck and at the top of your shoulders, if your neck hurts and the pain radiates to the shoulders. But don't use the ice pack on the upper and mid neck itself. The reason for this is that the neck is very sensitive to cold. The neck muscles tend to spasm when ice is applied to it, putting ice on the upper neck can even cause muscle rigidity. For example. If you have radiating pain that originates from your neck and travels down into your shoulder or arm. This radiating pain is caused by disc pressure in the area of the brachial nerve plexus. This plexus is found from the 5th cervical down to the 1st thoracic vertebra in your upper back (*not* upper neck). One of the characteristics of disc pressure is swelling, which is always relieved by cold or ice. So if you have radiating pain in the arm or shoulder from the neck, apply an ice pack on the lower portion of the neck, while avoiding placing it on the mid or upper portions of the neck. Put ice on for 20 minutes up to 4 times per day. Important: Don't fall asleep with the ice pack or use it for too long because you can cause an ice burn to happen (more is not always better).

Where else can ice be applied? You can put ice anywhere from the upper back where the neck meets the shoulders all the way down to the sacrum; again, using ice for 20 minutes up to 4 times per day. If you have radiating low back pain into the buttock, you can apply ice to the low back. But putting ice on your leg for radiating low back pain will not help. It is too far from the source of pain. For ice to work it needs to be applied to the source of the pain, not in the area where it is radiating to, which means you will have to place the ice somewhere in the spinal region because radiating pain is caused by a swollen disc.

USING HOT PACKS

When they should or should not be used? I recommend hot packs for home use. They do sell some "moist heat" packs, but the moisture in them is just not enough to do a lot of good. Hydroculator packs, the old fashioned hot pack used in therapy and chiropractic offices, are the best. The reason for this is the moisture that "pushes" the heat deep into the body. Without the moisture, hot electric pads only heat the surface (the skin) but do not heat into the body. A hydroculator pack will push the heat 10 times further into the body than a heating pad without moisture. You can buy hydroculator packs cheaply and they will last a long time. You heat them up like spaghetti. Put them in a pan of boiling water for about 15 minutes. Wrap a towel around the pack before putting it on your body. The heat should last about 20 minutes. At this time you may remove the pack. Use the pack up to 4 times a day.

Do not use heat on any areas of radiating pain. Why? Because when pain radiates down the arm or leg, a swollen disc causes it. What does heat do? It relieves muscle spasms; it sedates the nerves, but it also CAUSES swelling! So be careful. When you have disc pain radiating into your buttock and down your leg, you don't want more swelling in the problem disc area. It will feel good when the heat is on, but later it will feel much worse. Hot tubs and baths are the same. If you have just *minor* muscle fatigue and stiffness, hot tubs and baths are great! But for a swollen disc, they are not good and will likely make you hurt later. You may not even feel it until the next day. So when you use heat, make sure that there is no radiating pain associated with your injury. The hydroculator packs can be applied from the back of the head and neck down to the sacrum and on the buttocks.

Other things you can use at home include a trigger point cane (or thera cane) to put pressure on a muscle spasm. Pushing something into a muscle to relieve the spasm is usually fine, unless the pain radiates from that spot. Remember, again, if you have radiation of pain, you have a swollen disc. Don't force a thera cane into an area of a swollen disc. It may become worse later.

Hot tubs and baths

Living in Japan for several years taught me the wonderful effects of taking a very hot bath. The Japanese designed O'furo (Japanese bath) allows your entire body to be enveloped in lovely hot water. This warms up your entire body and all your muscles. I found that it decreased general back pain and body aches a great deal. Using the O'furo everyday makes you sleep better at night (hot water increases the para-sympathetic nervous system), and helps you feel better the next day! I must mention that for those experiencing low back pain that radiates into the buttocks or legs not to use heat because these symptoms are indicative of a swollen disc. Heat makes swelling worse, so be careful with heat. Hot tubs can be used like an O'furo, the only difference is that the water is chemically treated and they are often not as hot as the Japanese O'furo.

Hanshin Yoku

This is an old Japanese remedy for a myriad of problems. Try filling up the water in your tub to a level just above your belly button in a sitting position. Warming up the legs causes the upper body to warm more slowly, this process helps change your body constitution if done on a regular basis. Changing your body constitution means changing problems you may have like high blood pressure or heart problems. Hanshin yoku is very good for circulation and detoxification. Doing hanshin yoku will cause you to sweat. There are two kinds of sweat, one is a watery sweat and the other is a sticky sweat. Hanshin yoku causes you to emit a sticky sweat. Toxins come out with a sticky sweat. Before stepping into the tub, you should drink water because hanshin yoku can cause you to dehydrate some. You should do hanshin yoku for about 20 to 30 minutes, however, for some, hanshin yoku can take a few days to get use to, so monitor yourself to not get over done in the bath tub.

Massage

What about massage? Getting a massage is a wonderful thing and is a huge benefit for lifestyle and relaxation. Massage is usually good anywhere in the body, except in the low back when disc swelling and pressure exist. In the neck and shoulders, even if there is radiating pain and disc pressure, massage is generally all right. But in the low back, the discs are bigger, and massaging those areas of disc pressure and pain can irritate and even inflame the area more. If you do choose to get a massage while experiencing radiating low back pain, ask the massage therapist not to massage the low back. They may massage the buttocks area and down the legs and also massage the upper back down to about the mid back, but not the low back musculature. Remember, your condition can worsen if you choose to let them massage your low back while having a bout of low back pain. So grade yourself before getting a massage. If you are at a pain level of 0 to 6, go ahead and get massaged. If you are at a pain level of 7 or above, you may get massaged but not in the area of low back disc involvement. This is extremely dangerous and could extend your recovery time from this injury another week or more.

Massage, however, can be a wonderful tool to help cover up the secondary soft spot written about earlier. Remember, the secondary soft spot is alive and well after a bout of severe spinal pain due to subluxation. As I mentioned earlier, exercise is the major tool I use to combat the secondary soft spot. Muscle memory is what is causing the secondary soft spot in the first place. The muscles in the area of subluxation allowed the vertebra in question to slide out of place into a posterior position. After realigning the subluxated vertebra, exercise can strengthen the muscles in the area of the subluxation and basically cause the muscle memory to forget. In the area of subluxation, some muscles are over taught and act to "pull" the realigned vertebra out of place again. With massage, you can have a deep tissue, stripping massage to the over taught muscles, lengthening them and making them more supple. This can be accomplished in 3 to 5 treatments and actually works fantastic in conjunction with exercise.

Arch supports and orthotics

Arch supports are an often-overlooked way to help alleviate back pain. Have you ever noticed either on yourself or on other people, the big toe on either the right or left foot turns in at a sharper angle than the other big toe? There is usually a large knot at the base of the big toe when this has occurred. This knot is caused by degeneration. This condition where the arch drops and the arch flattens out causing the big toe to turn in is called Pes Planus, and is a degenerative situation caused by the dropping of the arch in the problem foot. An estimated 20 to 30 percent of the population is affected. It can also cause knee pain and hip pain for that matter. To slow the process down, those affected by this malady have to support the arch as much as possible. That means if you have this problem, you should not wear thongs! In Hawaii, where I live, thongs or slippers as we call then, are a way of life! To support the arch, one needs to where good tennis shoes or, better yet, running shoes. As far as athletic shoes, usually running shoes have a better arch support than other types of athletic shoes. Also the better the shoe, the more expensive the shoe will be. Other solutions are to buy good arch supports. Yes, some you can even glue into your thongs! Getting a good arch support is not easy, though. Getting an arch support that not only supports you but that feels good is sometimes hard to find. One solution is to order orthotics which are usually made to your foot. You step into a foam box that makes an imprint of your foot, then your orthotics are made from this model. The problem is that these expensive orthotics are usually hard and uncomfortable. You can ask your podiatrist or chiropractor if they have orthotics that are comfortable and supportive at the same time. These orthotics usually cost in the neighborhood of from 200 to 400 dollars. OUCH! But for many folks they are a lifesaver. Another solution is to order ready made orthotics, they are usually much cheaper and some are quite good.

Another treatment of pes planus is to make the foot more flexible. People with Pes Planus who have flexible feet develop fewer symptoms. Getting your feet to be more flexible is possible using the Chibi Ball. You can do so by either sitting in a chair or standing. Place the ball of your foot on the Chibi Ball and push the heel down, creating a stretch in the bottom of the foot for a few minutes. Then step directly on the chibi ball pushing the ball into the arch area and rolling it around a bit. If you repeat this about three or four times a week , you can help prevent pain from falling arches. If you have severe pain at the bottom of your foot, this may also be due to plantar fascitis. A condition when the fascia at the bottom of the foot between the ball of your foot and the heel is painful and actually hurts when you try to stretch the arch. What you need to do is soak the foot in hot water and Epsom salts and then massage the bottom of the foot. Then start stretching the arch of your foot using the chibi ball as described above. Also having the soles of your foot deeply massaged can help "break up" the irritated fascia.

Another frequently seen problem in my office is pain at the heel or in the arch of the foot caused by a bone spur. The bone spur grows from the heel towards the center of the foot. The bone spur is usually short and hook like. It can often cause a very deep heel pain. It's easy to diagnose however, just take an x-ray and your doctor can visualize it immediately. The cure for this is often surgery, but wearing soft support shoes is another solution, this will help you not to irritate the spur and the soft tissue surrounding it.

If you have foot problems, try going to a foot reflexologist! Reflexologists are trained not only in massaging the entire foot but also how some painful areas in the foot relate to other organs and problems in the body. It's very fascinating and this art has been around a long time. By the way, it can be very relaxing not to mention addicting!

Traction

Using various traction devices at home can also be useful in not only relieving neck or low back pain, but also it can be helpful in making your neck and low back healthier as we get older. Why do we become shorter when we get older? The biggest reason for this is because our discs loose their height and fluid content as we get older. Traction can help this loss of disc height to slow down. Traction lengthens the spine and helps the imbibition process talked about earlier in the book.

Good traction devices for low back are the inversion tables and the traction "pump" devices. The inversion tables are very stable and allow you to lean back and get the desired stretch you want. The kind of inversion table that's best is the one with the full length table, not one that hangs you by your knees. Also don't use the old method of hanging from gravity boots. When you hang straight down from gravity boots, there is a shear force that can occur in the lumbar area causing sudden severe pain.

The traction pump devices are new and allow you to "pump up" the device with a blood pressure kind of device. It works well and you can really feel it! They are also fairly cheap. Both the inversion table and the pump traction devices mentioned here are not helpful for the cervical region.

Cervical traction devices are basically in two types:

One is the cervical pump unit, again using a blood pressure type device to inflate it with air that expands the unit and tractions your neck. I have used these in my clinics and most patients liked them. Some patients felt a slight constriction around the neck, making it difficult to breath. The other more difficult device used for cervical traction is the over the door unit. It attaches to the top of the door. You sit in a chair with a harness around your head and a water filled bag, used for weight, tractions your neck. These devices have been used for years and work well. They are cheap but are harder to set up every time you want to use them. The choice is yours.

CHAPTER FOUR

....

Ergonomics in Daily Life

You might have thought there were more at home things to do to relieve back pain, but the truth is that it is better to avoid getting back pain altogether. Ergonomics at home and in the office are the most important aspects in prevention. If you can make good posture a habit in all areas of your life, your back will feel so much better all the time. Let's start off with posture. Standing posture is so important for two reasons.

One reason is that, believe it or not, standing in a proper posture helps give you a positive attitude. For example, which posture makes you feel more confident, slouching with your head down or when your head is held high and your shoulders are squared? The mind is affected by our posture for sure. Try walking down the hall with your head held low and your shoulder curled forward. See how you feel. I'll bet you'll notice a depressed feeling right away. Now try the opposite. Try walking with your head held high and your shoulders erect and square. I'll bet you will notice an immediate change in your attitude! A positive feeling!

The second reason is that standing in correct posture is good for your spine. Essentially, a correct posture is keeping the spine in the proper position for which it was designed.

So *what* exactly is the proper posture?
Walk over to an unobstructed wall. Stand with your heels as well as your buttocks against it. Now, let your upper back and shoulder area touch the wall. Finally put the back of your head against the wall. Feel this posture. For most of you, especially females, you may think that you are sticking your chest out too much. This, however, is proper posture.

I've heard Tai Chi practitioners say to tuck your pelvis under a bit is a better posture. This is not true. Tucking your pelvis will eventually injure your low back. You have a natural 35-degree curve in your low back for a reason. The reason is this: All the anatomical structures are made to accommodate this degree curve. End of story! From the ears, through the shoulders and pelvis, and down to the heels, everything lines up in a position of strength. If you don't allow a natural curve in your low back, you will have unnatural results: Subluxation. Tucking the pelvis under is an activity that is part of Tai Chi, Chi Quong, Pilates, and Yoga. But it is done for only a few moments. It is an exercise, if you will, and should never be done as part of your "normal" posture.

Let's now consider proper posture as it pertains to walking. The same posture should be maintained. Your head should be up, but if you will note that when leaning back against the wall, your head is up while your chin is slightly tucked. This is a natural position for standing, but don't walk around with your eyes or head looking up in the air. Your eyes should be looking straightforward. Your feet should land on the ground, heel to toe, while, of course, moving the arms naturally.

I've read many websites on how to walk properly. Many suggest you tuck in your tailbone while walking. Again, this is not a natural posture, it decreases the natural 35 degree lordodic curve in the lumbar spine. I personally don't know why many "experts" in the field suggest doing something which is not only un-natural but detrimental to the spine and lumbar discs. Even a pain free "normal" spine would start to have problems in a short amount of time if an individual were to walk around like this. I have had many a patient come in with severe disc injuries due to just this abnormal walking procedure that they were told to do by an "expert".

Now about sitting: The sitting position is where you will put the most load on the lumbar discs. Sitting should be done like standing. You will retain your natural low back curve (not extreme curve, but your natural curve). If you sit and accentuate your low back curve too much, you will cause too much muscle tension in this area. So sit down with your low back almost straight or a slight lordodic curve present.

Now an important point: While sitting down, your knees should be positioned out a bit. Although sitting with your knees together is proper in our society, having the knees out slightly is much better on the low back. It creates a strong, more stable sitting position. Also it does not put pressure on the hip joints in this position, which happens when you sit with your knees together. Now, from a sitting position, you may lean back in a chair to relax. There are two ways to do this. One is to lean back putting a firm pillow behind your low back, which should be hard enough to push back on your lumbar curve and provide support. You may lean back this way for hours because it will give the support you need. The other way is to just lean back without a pillow, while keeping your natural lumbar curve. It can be done as long as the chair you are leaning against is hard enough to press

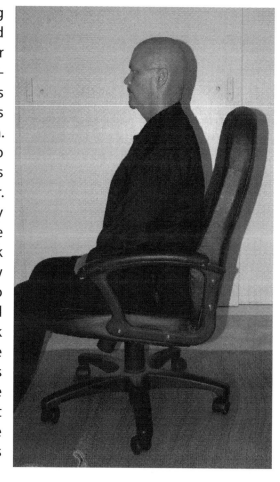

against with your upper back. I do this in my computer chair. I can stay like this for hours with no discomfort whatsoever. The reason I can do this is because I'm keeping my low back curve, and I am doing this using my own muscular tension.

In review, what causes back pain? Subluxation. What causes subluxation? Flexion of the spine. Why is flexion capable of causing subluxation? Because the vertebrae don't move forward or anterior --they can only move backward (posterior). Does flexion of the spine always cause the vertebrae to move backward, resulting in sub-luxation? No. Flexion of the spine in a controlled environment is done deliberately, like yoga, stretching, or working out at the gym. It is done to stretch and lengthen the muscles associated with the low back. This is good flexion. Remember, we talked about degeneration? What causes the spine to degenerate? It is non-movement of the spine in a certain area. Why does this cause degeneration? The discs receive nutrition, not through the circulatory system like most areas of our bodies, but by a squeezing motion of the spine. It is called imbibition, which happens when the spine is moved around. Imbibition is a good thing. That's why exercise and yoga are good. But in the office and at home in daily life, sitting wrong can severely injure your low back. Yet sitting improperly is not the only way to injure your back. Any improper flexing of the spine from the low back all the way up to the neck can cause back problems.

What is one to do then?

First things first, let's start with the office. The most important equipment as it per-tains to your back, is the chair you sit in. The chair must support your low back. There are some exceptions to this, but let's consider your chair first. The chair should be at the proper height and position to allow you to place both feet firmly on the floor. The chair should have a low back support that pushes into your mid lumbar spine where your natural curve is. The exceptions to this are two things. First, if you are accustomed to keeping your own spine slightly arched all the time, you won't need a chair to push into your low back. The second exception about chairs is the seat itself. The seat should be cushy. If it is too hard, a chair that pushes into the back of the thighs and butte can irritate, even bruise the tailbone. Once this occurs, it can be quite painful and can take a long time to heal. The other thing that can happen is the back of the thighs can be compressed. If this happens, it can upset the sciatic nerve coming from the low back down the legs, causing the back of the thighs to be achy, but, more importantly, it can also irritate the sciatic nerve making the pain travel down to the calves and feet. This can happen sitting in your car as well. It's called driving sciatica and results from pressure against the back of your thighs caused by your seat cushion putting pressure on the back of your thighs.

When sitting on your chair at the office, it is not always necessary to sit straight up. I always lean back in my chairs and keep my arch naturally, as I mentioned before. Holding the spine too straight, too upright, can cause your back to feel tired when you're not use to it. Leaning back can make the back muscles relaxed, but do not ever slouch. Slouching is one of the number-one causes of disc injuries in the low back. Slouching is never good and should never be done. Many of my patients in their 20's still slouch when they sit. They also have back pain (not surprisingly). At some point in their lives, they will have to stop slouching because of their own increasing low back pain. It does teach you a lesson not to slouch once you have had a severe bout of low back pain. Also, while sitting in the chair, you should look straight into the computer monitor; don't turn your head all day looking at the screen sideways for obvious reasons. Also your desk height should be optimum for you. You should not have to hold your shoulders high up because of having the chair too low or the table too high. The height should be comfortable where your elbows hang from your shoulders and arms resting comfortably on top of the table.

Ergonomics at Home

Ergonomics at home is even more important than ergonomics at the office. At home you lounge more than you do at work (hopefully -- unless you have a job we're all looking for!). When sitting at home on the computer, you should follow the same rules mentioned above for the office. Sitting on a couch can be brutal on your back because you can slouch for hours watching a movie. For sitting on a couch you can sit two ways; some prefer to sit straight up, having a cushion supporting the lumbar curve, while others prefer lying back with a cushion supporting the lumbar curve. Note that both positions require a lumbar support. This lumbar support should be thick enough to really support the low back. In other words, if you have a little belly, it should pop it out a bit. (Although none of us have a belly like that!)

Lying and sitting on the floor is okay, too. The important thing is to move around; don't lie in one position for hours at a time. While living in Japan, I noticed that people born and raised there sit with their backs very straight. They also have good flexibility. They can sit crossed legged and squat down on their haunches with no problems at all. But sitting on the floor putting a newspaper in front of you and bending to read it is not a good thing; it causes the low back curve to move into flexion.

Reading in bed is another potential hazard. Don't prop your head on a pillow to look down at your book, because this will hold your head in a flexed position. Holding this for hours will definitely cause problems in your neck. The same thing goes for propping the head up in bed to look at a TV in the bedroom. It will prove to be a bad decision, one of those we often make without thought at the time – only to reap the negative consequences later on. So when watching TV or reading in bed, you should put two, three or four pillows behind you, starting at the low back and continuing up your back, finishing with a pillow behind your head. The point to remember is to not flex the spine, especially the neck and low back. You can read like this for hours without pain or possibility of subluxation. They do have beds that adjust electronically into a more ergonomic position for watching TV and for reading in bed. (Expensive!)

Beds

Having the right bed is extremely important! Memory foam beds have become quite popular these days. I find them very comfortable and supportive at the same time. They come in a variety of styles and firmness. Other more traditional beds are also good. They should be firm and hold their shape, which usually means they are going to be on the expensive side to buy. But you spend almost one third of your life in bed, so it's wise to spend more to get a better bed.

The only drawback to memory foam beds is that they give off quite a bit of gases from the foam. It does dissipate as the mattress gets older but for some it may cause a problem. The best way to experiment with this problem is to buy a memory foam pillow and sleep on it for a while. If gases bother you from the pillow, then for sure the memory foam mattress will bother you too. I also recommend traditional Japanese futons. Not the American hybrid futons. The popular American models don't hold their shape and are generally too soft. The problem is that they are too thick and soft. A Japanese futon is thin, about 3 inches thick. That means you can slightly feel the floor underneath you. Japanese futons are really meant to be on top of a tatami mat, which is used for traditional flooring in Japan and are made of woven grass. They are softer than hardwood, so when your futon is on top of tatami mat, it's very comfortable. I prefer the firmness.

Generally I have found that sleeping on a very firm mattress is better for people with low back problems. While those folks who have upper back or neck problems need a medium firm mattress. If you are in extreme low back pain, over a 7 on a 1 to 10 scale, you should try sleeping a few nights on the floor. You can sleep on a few sleeping bags or two layers of mattress pads to give your sore back support. Once your pain level drops below a 7, you can start to sleep on your firm bed again. This is only a suggestion.

Engaging your Butt!

Let's talk about doing the ordinary routines of life, such as washing dishes, brushing your teeth, or vacuuming. All these mundane activities are done while engaging your butt (or buttocks, if you prefer). Example: Stand, sticking your butt out a little, increasing your arch in your low back. Now, bend your knees a bit and you will not hurt your back while doing these chores. Believe it or not, these daily activities cause you to slightly flex the spine if done without bending the knees and engaging your buttocks. A five-degree forward bend is actually loading the spine with a lot more pressure than you realize. It can lead to disc problems and subluxation. If you have ever had a low back pain when you sneezed or coughed (indicative of a disc injury), bending over to brush your teeth can be very painful.

Lifting

Lifting is very similar. Have you ever seen a power lifter? Before they engage in lifting weights, they always prepare first by sticking their butt out and bending their knees. This puts the low back in a strengthened position. Remember, we have this low back curve for a reason. Now that you know spinal anatomy, you also know that the low back curve helps protect your body. Before lifting anything, remember to stick your butt out and bend your knees as you get close to the item that you intend to lift. Bend yours knees (not your back!) as you get your hands under the item and lift by straightening your knees while keeping the low back arched. You will not hurt your low back in this way. The challenge in lifting this way, however, is if you have bad knees. Lifting properly with bad knees can be difficult. In fact, it may be impossible to lift this way, but if you must lift without bending the knees due to a knee problem, then lift only light items or get help.

Another good thing to do is to wear a lumbar support. If you have ever had a low back pain that was fairly severe, you know that coughing or even going to the bathroom makes it worse, much worse. Moreover, if you have had pain down the leg (sciatica), when going to the bathroom, the pain down the leg increases with the amount of push you try to muster. What causes this? The cause is interthecal pressure, which is the thecal sack that surrounds the spinal cord swelling slightly whenever you hold your breath and push. When I examine a patient whom I suspect to have a disc injury, I have him hold his breath and push as if he were going to the bathroom. In doing this, if he has a sharp increase in pain, it is due to the thecal sac touching a protruding or swollen disc. This evaluating maneuver is called Valsalva's test. It indicates a disc protrusion, if the patient exhibits a positive Valsalva's test. I have the patient take an MRI. Usually the MRI will show some kind of disc problem, ranging from a disc protrusion, which can get better with treatment, or a herniated disc, which can also improve with treatment (using the Kiso Method instead of twisting the lumbar spine while adjusting), though it is much more severe. A herniated disc means the disc has ripped. Once you have a disc that is damaged in this way, it will always be damaged. Does it mean you have to have surgery? Not always, but sometimes it is a consideration. How would a disc herniation come about? SUBLUXATION! How can I help cure a subluxation? ADJUST THE SPINE!

So, getting back to my reference earlier about lumbar supports, make sure that it is a 9 or 10 inch wide support. Also use what is called a double pull support. Once you wrap the lumbar support around you, you pull additional straps, one on each side to further tighten the support. These straps pull in the middle of the support slightly arching your lumbar curve slightly. With this type of support all the low back muscles are supported. It will also keep the low back in a more proper position, not allowing it to flex and bend easily. Thus, a vertebra with a swollen or damaged disc will have a harder time pushing itself into the thecal sac of the spinal cord. If the disc does touch the thecal sac of the spinal cord, it sets off an almost "electrical" quality of pain. This pain can either be local to the low back or it can travel down the sciatic nerve. So remember to wear a wide double pull support whenever you lift. Although the supports for weight lifting also help, most are not wide enough.

Also wearing a tight small leather belt can cause back pain when the belt constantly pushes on an injured disc or subluxated area.

Other chores around the house include weeding and outside work as well as cleaning the bathtub, sink, floors, and so on – all "back breakers" aren't they? Or are they? For example, if you learn proper positioning, you can initially have a sore low back, weed for an hour, and even feel better afterwards! The reason for this is while weeding you have engaged your butt. This causes a warming up of the muscles in the low back region without further injuring the subluxation that originally made your back sore. Also by doing this activity properly you actually strengthen the legs and low back, which, in turn, help to stabilize your entire back.

CHAPTER FIVE

....

Stabilizing Exercises

In regards to back pain, there is a reason for exercising first and stretching afterwards. The order is important. When an individual has a disc problem, your back is vulnerable to injury – and stretching can be one of those mechanisms of injury. But how do you know you have a disc problem? Besides having an MRI that confirms the problem, you may have one of the following:

1) Pain upon taking a deep breath and pushing when using the restroom (Valsalva's Test).
2) Pain traveling down into the buttocks, down the legs, and in the calf or the foot. This pain can be felt on either side or both.
3) Weakness or tingling in the buttocks, legs or feet.
4) Sharp severe pain in the low back that is almost electric in feeling. This may be accompanied by strong muscle spasms in the low back region.
5) Constant muscle spasm around the spine, buttocks or reoccurring spasm in the upper and lower legs.

If you have any of the above, you are not ready for stretching yet! You must go to your Kiso practitioner or chiropractor and get adjusted first.

The Secondary soft spot

When a vertebra is subluxated, it is misaligned. When a chiropractor adjusts it, your vertebra is realigned into its "old seat", if you will. This old seat that we push the vertebra back into is called the primary soft spot. When you have a subluxated vertebra, there is a primary soft spot waiting for it to return. Once realigned, however, there is also a compensatory secondary soft spot, which the subluxation had created (the spot where the vertebra had misaligned into). Have you ever heard of muscle memory? Muscle memory is the primary reason for this secondary soft spot. When a vertebra is out of place, the reason it is out of place is due to the fact that the muscles, ligaments, and tendons that hold the vertebra in place have softened and have allowed it to move or misalign. So when you have a realigned vertebra, it is happily back into the primary soft spot, nicely getting used to its old proper position – and that would be the end of the story, if there was not a secondary soft spot waiting for the vertebra to slip back into!

When you have had a bout with back pain from subluxation, the process of "holding" the adjustment can sometimes be frustrating for the patient, who has to return continuously for readjustments for vertebrae that keep slipping out of place. Some people give up on chiropractors because of this. They get disillusioned – "Yea, the adjustment feels great right afterwards, but then – wham! This is all due to the secondary soft spot. This scenario is very common, and repeated (and repeated) visits can be a very expensive for the patient. How do you cover up the secondary soft spot and make it disappear?

Exercise!

Exercise is the primary weapon we have for this. Exercise will strengthen the muscles and the tendons. Tendons are either the origin of the muscle in question or the insertion of the muscle. So when you strengthen the muscle, you also strengthen the tendons, both of which hold the vertebra in the realigned position. The reason the pain is coming back is usually due to a few factors. The biggest factor may be that your sitting position in the car is improper. You may have allowed your low back to be in a flexed position while driving.

Another factor is that your muscles and tendons were not toned enough to hold the adjustment in place. Generally, when a patient comes in with severe low back pain, it will be weeks before I recommend exercise. If the patient is an athlete, exercises can be done sooner than for those who have never exercised before. Before exercising though, I want to make sure the subluxation is fixed. It may take several adjustments per week to get the job done.

Once the patient feels much better, I recommend exercises. I have the patient start first with exercises that are not likely to cause the subluxation to occur. The exercises are graded from I to III. The grading is simple. On a scale of 1 to 10, 10 being the worst pain, where do you fall in? 0 to 2 is a grade I. 3 to 6 is a grade II. A grade 7 and above is grade III, which is called an acute stage. Doing exercises as soon as possible is the key to truly stabilizing the patient's back. But you don't want to begin too early, because not only will it not help stabilize your back, it may even raise the pain scale closer to a 10. Now keep in mind, the exercises below are stabilizing exercises. They are not meant for aerobic use; rather, they are to maintain your low back to be "subluxation-free".

Let's now look at the exercises

Remember Grade III means you are at a pain level of from 7 to 10. This means you are in a lot of pain. Grade II means you're at a pain level of between 3 and 6. This means you are in moderate pain. Grade I means you are at a pain level of between 0 and 2. This means you have no pain or only slight pain.

GRADE III
You should not exercise. You need to heal more and get to a pain level of 6 or below.

GRADE II

You still have moderate pain but can do some stabilizing exercises.
The stabilizing exercises below are suitable for grade II and grade I people.

"Supermans": Lying face down, put your arms out in front of you and raise your arms up off the floor while also raising your legs off the floor. This makes the muscles in the buttocks and lumbar area work.

Note: Do not bend your knees; you must keep the legs straight as you raise them off the floor from the buttocks. Hold each repetition about two seconds and do what's comfortable for you (usually from 10 to 60 depending on your condition).

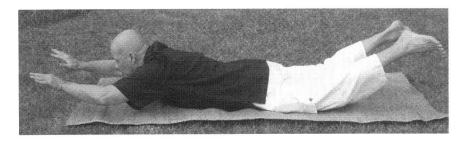

"Scissors": Still lying face down, you can either keep your arms out in front of you or you can keep them under your chest. Now lift both legs up off the floor from the buttocks and once your legs are out straight behind you, cross your feet with your toes pointed. At first it feels difficult to do more than 8 or 10, but in a week's time you will be doing 20 to 50. They are very beneficial for the sacrum and the pelvis.

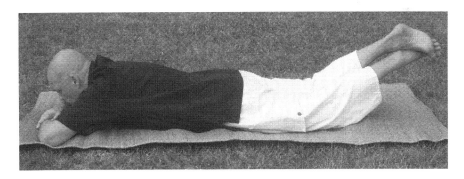

"Forward crunches": Lying face up with your knees bent, fold your arms in front of your chest. Raise your chest and head up off the floor by "shortening" your abdominal muscles. You don't need to lift your entire torso off the ground like an old-fashion sit up, which are harmful for the low back. It's a good idea to keep your face and eyes looking up toward the ceiling while doing this exercise. This will ensure that you don't flex the neck too much. Now hold each repetition about two seconds. Do as many as you are comfortable doing. Try and do two sets of between 10 and 35.

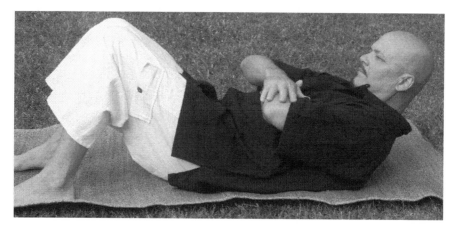

GRADE I

You can do the exercises above, plus the following.

"Side crunches": Lie on your back on the floor with your knees up.
Turn facing your knees to one side, while keeping your chest and head flat on the floor. Lift your upper torso up off the floor as you did with the crunches. Each repetition should be held about two seconds. Now do the other side.

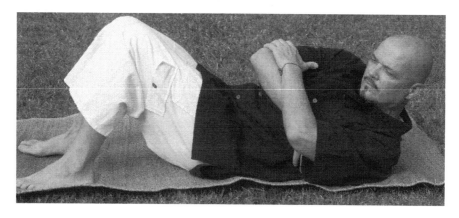

"Wall squats": Find a clear area on a wall at home. Slide down the wall bending your knees with your feet shoulder-width apart. Go down to where your knee bends at about a 90-degree angle. Once in this position, now push up to a standing position and then go back down again. You can do as many as you are comfortable. Do them slowly.

"Ball sit ups": Using a big rubber exercise ball, sit on it while bending your knees and placing your toes under something for support. Now do sit ups by leaning back about half way and then pulling yourself up again back to a sitting position. Do as many as you like. These are more strenuous than crunches.

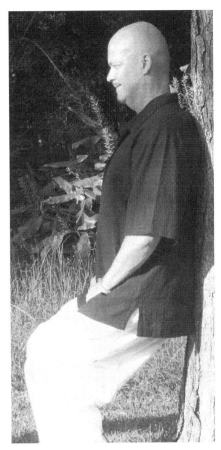 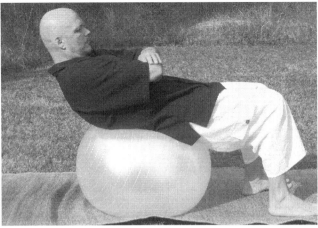

"Ball back ups": With a big rubber ball again, lay across it with your hips and stomach centered on top. Put your legs outstretched behind you and under something for support or have someone hold your legs. Now bend over the ball with your hands behind your head or your hands held at your chest. Holding your hands behind your head is more difficult. Raise yourself up arching your back slightly at the top of the movement. Do as many as you are comfortable with.

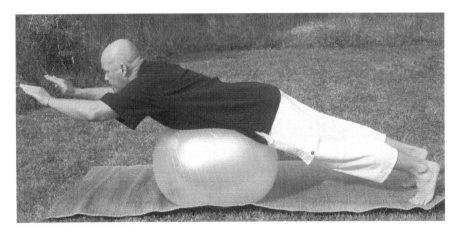

"Kick backs": On all fours on the floor, kick back the right leg. Kick the leg straight out behind you, all the way to slightly up at full extension. Now do the other leg. You can do up to 30 on each side.

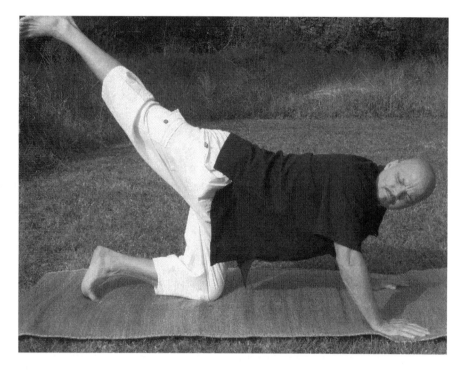

"Cat backs": On all fours, lift your head while sticking your butt out and creating an arch in your back. Hold for two seconds. Now do the opposite. Tuck your head down while arching your low back up and tucking your butt under. Hold for two seconds. You can do 10 to 20.

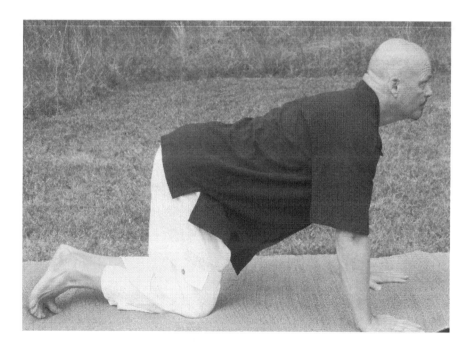

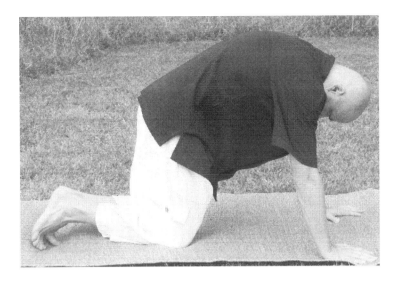

"Side raises": On all fours, lift your bent leg on the right up as high as you can. Now repeat on the other side. Do as many as are comfortable.

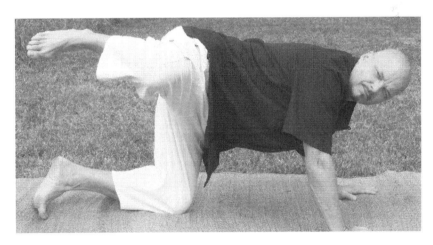

"Pelvic thrusts": Laying face up on the floor with your knees up, keep your arms at your side resting on the floor for stability. Now raise the hips up as far as you can off the floor. Do between 10 and 30. You can do these rather fast, in a rather continuous fashion.

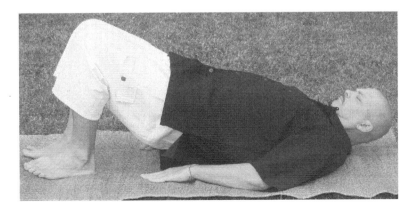

"Lunges".

Standing with feet shoulder width apart, step forward. Your front knee should be bent at a 90 degree angle with your foot pointing straight ahead. As you step make sure you extend out. Once your foot is on the floor in front of you, now you will bring that same foot back again to the starting position. Now step out with the other foot. You may do up to 10 or 12 repetitions. This exercise can be used with small weights in your hands, hanging down at your sides. This exercise is great for conditioning the buttocks and thighs.

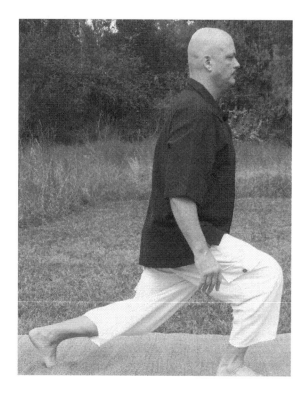

Core Exercises

Building strength in your core muscles is simple and easy. Many disciplines, such as Yoga, Pilates etc., incorporate core strengthening exercises into their routines. I am going to recommend three moves to quickly strengthen your core muscles and help maintain your spinal strength. These exercises can be done about 3 or 4 times a week to maintain core strength.

1. Lay face down on the floor and raise yourself into a push-up position, keeping your legs and waist as straight as you can. Hold this position for one minute breathing in and out through the nose.

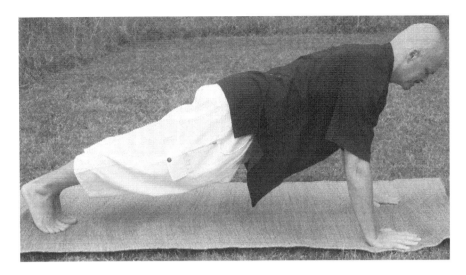

2. Now, keeping your feet where they were in the number 1 position and maintaining the straight legs and waist, turn your body sideways. As you do this raise your arm high toward the ceiling. Hold for one minute breathing naturally through the nose.

Now rotate to the other side and hold for one minute.

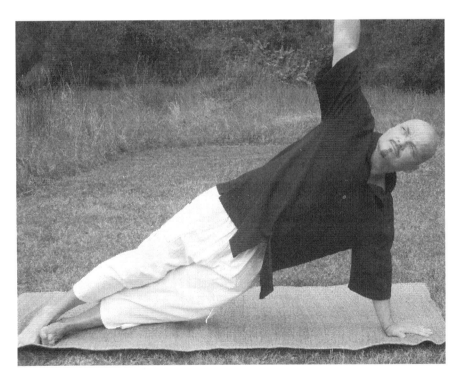

3. Now turn face-up with your arms holding you rigid and keeping your legs and waist in a straight line. Hold one minutes breathing naturally through the nose.

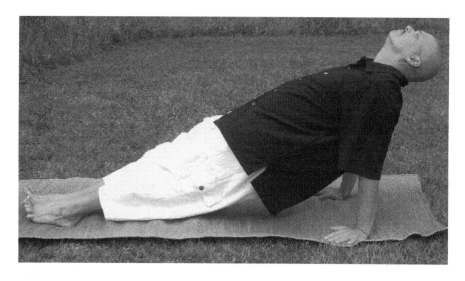

Machine exercises for Grade I and II are found usually in gyms. Not every gym has them. If you don't have access to a gym, then the ball sit-ups and ball back-ups are great! The only difference is that the machines found in the gym can allow you more resistance if you are so inclined and are more on the athletic side. I include them here because many

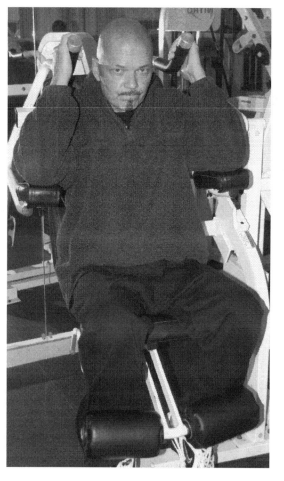

patients ask me what are the best exercising machines found in gyms as well as the worst. The machines that are best for stabilizing the low back are simple. Either the machine will provide resistance for the low back or for the abdominal muscles in the stomach. These machines only move the body forward or backward. They do not move your body in any other direction. If you see a piece of equipment in a gym that is designed to make you turn at the waist, do not use this piece of equipment! Turning while adding weight is a bad idea and can injure you. Another good machine is the one used for doing squats that has a good strong seat for supporting the back. The reason I include this piece of athletic equipment is due to the fact that this machine helps build the gluteal muscles which are essential for stabilizing the back. You can actually put a rolled up small towel behind your low back to slightly increase the lumbar curve for added support.

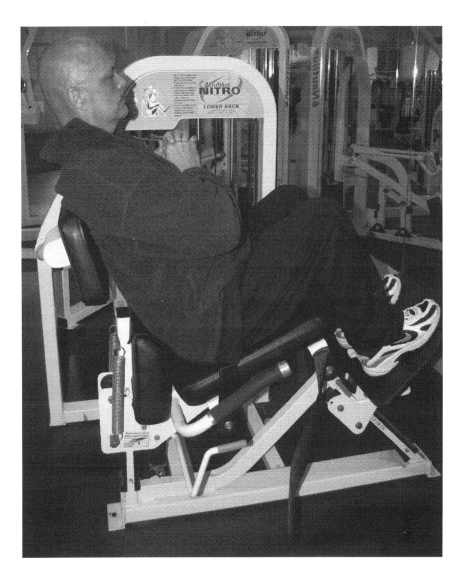

There is another apparatus, it's not really a machine. It's an apparatus which you can bend forward on, putting your pelvis over a pad and locking your legs and knees against another pad behind you. You may bend forward, flexing the spine and then pull back up using your low back extensor muscles. This apparatus in only recommended for grade I or grade II people. You may also hold a weight to increase resistance. With this apparatus, you can do 10 to 20 reps and do one to three sets.

I don't recommend any other machine. In particular, machines which force you to twist your waist against resistance are dangerous. Turning and loading the spine at the same time is asking for trouble. If you are a professional athlete, go ahead and do it, but if not, stick with the exercises above.

Yet with even the machines that I recommend for either the low back or the stomach muscles, first make sure that you are a grade I or a grade II, and, secondly, take it easy with the amount of weight or resistance. Also, don't move into flexion too deeply, meaning do not overextend or bend too far forward. For example, when pushing back against weight, keep your low back as straight as possible and don't round the low back before pushing. This will lessen the chance of hurting the low back. The same goes for doing the abdominal machines. Don't curl forward, rounding the low back, but try and keep the lumbar spine as straight as possible. You will still be able to do the exercises correctly. The amount of weight can easily reach two hundred pounds or more without injuring the spine (for women it might be less). Remember, your spine is made to push and pull with weight, however it is not meant for turning and twisting with weight. If you are used to doing yoga and do not usually use a weight machine, you might want to try weight resistance for stabilizing the low back.

The low back muscles are meant to cause the lumbar spine to curve into extension or lordosis. What allows the lumbar spine to move into a dangerous position called kyphosis (flexion) is the lack of tone in the lower back muscle. Tonus in the muscles only comes from working the muscle out in a particular way. At one end of the spectrum, the bodybuilder has extreme tonus. That means even when he or she is not pumping the muscles up, their muscles are slightly tense. On the other hand, if you have a person who never works out at all, your muscles will be flaccid (jellylike with no tonus). To contrast these two extremes, when walking around and working in daily life, the flaccid person will be the one to suffer from all kinds of subluxation due to the fact that there is no tonus in the muscles. Tonus helps hold the skeletal system together. Now please note that you can have a relaxed, beautiful body without being a bodybuilder. Just having a nice amount of tonus is all you need. Doing the above exercise 2 or 3 times a week will do the trick.

Your back is made to work. The low back is designed for heavy work. It does not mean we have to do heavy work but that is what it was designed for. If we don't work our backs, our backs will become weak and this will lead to subluxation. The exercises above may be viewed as light for many people, but they are all you need. You don't need convoluted and sophisticated back exercises, you just need to work the back, flexing and extending it, in order to strengthen it.

Note: Some folks have a hyper lordodic curve or too much curve in the low back. Try working out the abdominal muscles extra hard to compensate for this problem.

Upper back exercises

For those in a category of a grade 1 or grade 11, you can combat chronic tight muscles in the upper back and neck by doing the following exercises twice a day. These exercises are created to increase blood flow to these upper back and neck muscles.

Chronic tight muscles are painful due to a decrease in blood flow. Doing the following exercises while at work or at home should help a great deal.

BIRD EXERCISES

Stand or sit. Put arms out straight and do circles quickly forward and back. Do this for about 1 minutes. Continue breathing while performing these exercises. Now bend your arms at the elbows and do circles again both forward and backward with elbows pointing out.

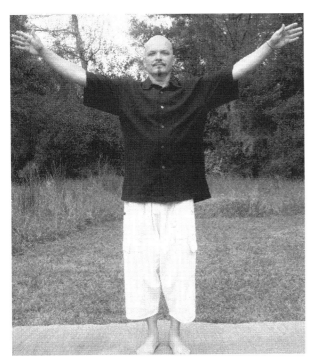
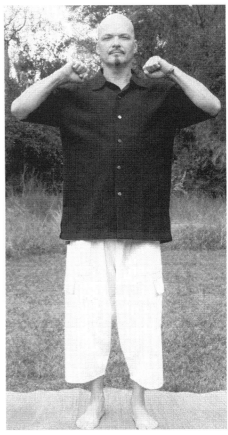

THE LOOK!

While standing, keep your waist straight, don't bend at the waist. You will bend in the upper back. Now, with your arms out at about a 45% angle. Look to the right and bring your right arm behind you with your left arm, coming across your body, following the right arm. While doing this exercise look to the right behind you. Do three to the right, then three to the left. The trick is this, as you are bending to the right look to the right. During your three movements, try and look behind you more each time. This will increase your flexibility each time you turn. You should feel this exercise between the shoulder blades. Do this three times on the right and three times on the left, doing three movements in each direction.

Tai Chi Drop

While standing, engage your buttocks and drop your knees slightly, about two inches. Now raise your arms above your head and in one swoop, drop your arms down, letting gravity take them down. At the same time, drop your knees and learn forward slightly. You are engaging your buttocks so it won't hurt your low back. As you go to the bottom, your hands will be close to the floor. Now raise up the arms above your head while extending your knee almost straight again. This is an excellent exercise, increasing blood flow to the entire body. Do this for one minute, breath in while raising your arms above your head and breath out when letting the arms drop.

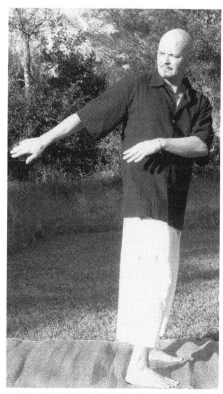

Gun Points

While standing, clasp your hands together, lacing your fingers into one another while pointing both your index fingers straight out together like a gun. Now, once in a neutral position, extend your fingers out about two inches further using the muscles in the upper back to force the arms and hands out in front of you. At the same time slightly rock your head back, engaging your muscles in the upper neck as well. Do about a minutes worth of these exercises.

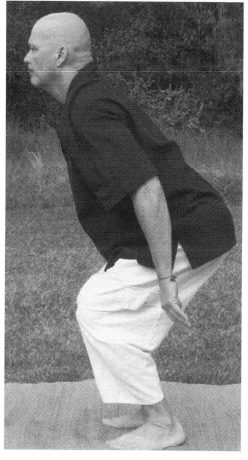

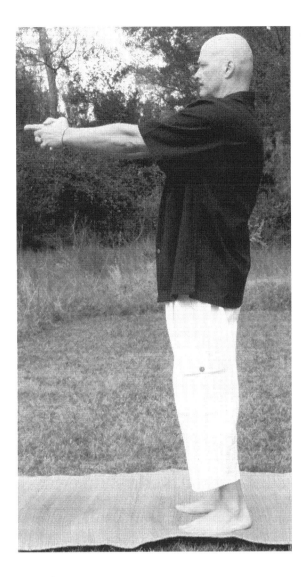

What else is good?

Now, in addition to those exercises, what else is good for the spine? Along with strengthening the low back you will also need to do some type of aerobic workout three or four time a week. These should be done for 20 to 40 minutes a day. You can do more but it's not necessary for keeping the body in great shape. Remember, stress comes in many forms. Stress is something that puts a load on the body as well as the mind. Many people get caught up in exercising too much and become stress junkies. I've seen them for years coming into my clinics. Yes, they may be in great shape but they are in the "fight or flight mode", which means that they often are easily agitated or anxious (or both!). This is not healthy for your mind or body. So if you want to do more, make sure you are doing more because you enjoy it. When exercise becomes a stress, it is not fun anymore. So be careful not to do too much. Too much means you are dreading it. If you are not the athletic type, then just do 20 minutes of some activity you enjoy, reaching your target heart rate while doing it. The low back exercises can take less than 5 minutes a day. You don't have to go nuts worrying about getting in great condition. I believe that it is better to keep your MIND in great condition than your body. So watch all the cues your mind and body are telling you and just relax and enjoy the process. As we will see in a later chapter, food will do as much in keeping your body in shape as exercise!

Note: They say that one mark of a true guru (teacher in the Indian tradition), is that a true guru is cheerful. I think that keeping your mind unencumbered and open is one key to longevity. So be open to new things. One proverb I've always thought was a truism was written by a true master (who, I don't know), it goes like this: The usefulness of the cup is in it's emptiness. I just love this! Don't keep your mind stiff and full, keep it empty and open!!

Aerobic Exercises

Again, grades are used to categorize the aerobic exercises that you may do. As the grades move from III to I, you will see that the exercises have more varied motions. The reason that walking is the only exercise in Grade III is because of the natural but limited amount of motion that is possible through walking, while swimming has much more twisting and turning. Even though swimming is a non-weight bearing exercise, it can re-injure those in a grade III situation.

GRADE III
Walking on level ground for short periods, about 5 to 20 minutes.
Remember Grade III means your pain level is a 7 or above. Walking on level ground will only be possible if you are at a 7 or 8. If your pain level in approaching a 9 or 10, don't do anything but rest and heal.

GRADE II
Walking on roads or on good trails for long periods should be fine.
But still avoid steep uphill walks because in order to go uphill, you must lean forward. This puts a strain on the lumbar spine and can cause the injured lumbar discs to become irritated. So try to avoid steep hills. You may also engage in the following aerobic exercises:

*Stair master
*Elliptical
*Treadmill (but avoiding steep uphill settings.)
*Swimming
*Pilates (only very easy moves, avoiding flexion of the spine.)

Grade II is when you are feeling better but still have some residual soreness. In this stage you can do many things: Walking up to one hour, walking on slightly uphill and down hill grades is usually OK, and swimming for 20 to 40 minutes is usually fine also. Swimming is sometimes hard on the neck, because of the rotation to breathe, and it can sometimes irritate the low back due to the twisting involved. That's why I don't recommend it for Grade III people. The stair master is usually good because it requires you to stick your butt out and arch your back. It is also great for working the gluteul muscles. Remember, these muscles are essential to building a strong back. The Elliptical machine is also good because it works the lower body without stressing the joints. The treadmill is effective only at a walking pace because running during a Grade II period can be harmful. The jarring movement that occurs while running can upset a healing disc. You can also do pilates, but avoid any moves that require flexing the low back and neck.

GRADE I

All of the above plus the following:

* Walking
* Swimming
* Stair master
* Elliptical
* Treadmill
* Pilates
* Dancing
* Jogging

Grade I means that your back is either healed or close to it. You can run up or down hills; walk up or down hills; swim to your hearts content; and you can also do pilates. Remaining in a Grade I should be your lifelong goal, and this can be achieved through ongoing exercising, proper lifting and posture, stretching (even Yoga), and diet, as will be discussed later in this book.

Aerobic Guidelines

Some guidelines for aerobic gain are the following:
* Work out at about 60 to 80 percent of your maximum heart rate rather than 85 or 90 percent. A faster heart rate is not better. You actually burn more fat at 60 percent of your heart rate than at 70 or 80 percent. To calculate your target working-out heart rate, minus your age from 220 and multiply this number by 60 for the low number, and then by 80 for the high number. Then you can stay between these two numbers. This will give you your target heart range. While running, you should be able to talk

and breathe without laboring this will mean you are still under 60 percent of your maximum heart rate. If you are breathing very hard and are unable to talk, you are probably above your target heart rate.

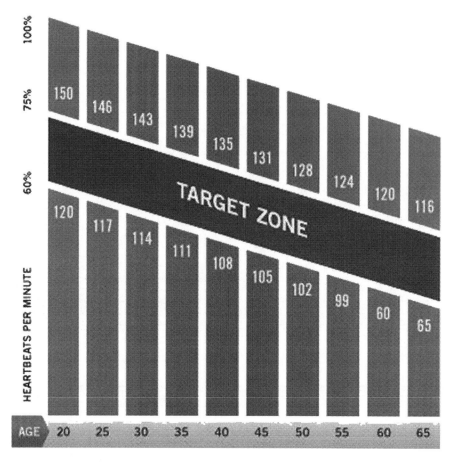

* Do aerobic activity early in the morning. It burns more fat (assuming you have not eaten a giant breakfast). But a cautionary note is that the older you are, the better it is to work out in the evening. This is due to the fact that your body is more warmed up and you will have fewer injuries. Working out in the morning right after waking up is sometimes hard on the muscles. You can sustain muscle and tendon injuries if you are not careful.

* The other cautionary note is to do your aerobic workouts with one day of rest in between. That way you have one day of rest to allow your muscles, tendons and joints to heal from the previous day. Cross training is key for any exercise routine. If, for example, you want to do six days of aerobic activity in one week, you should do three days of running every other day, and the stair master on the days in between, so you are not working out the same exact muscles every single day. Working the same exact muscles by doing the same activity six days a week will most certainly cause muscle and tendon problems. An ideal regime is to do three or four days of aerobic activity spaced apart by rest days in between. On the aerobic rest day, you

can do another activity such as weight lifting, yoga or some other completely different activity. It is also good for the psyche to mix things up to keep it interesting.
* Your aerobic activity should be preceded with a short stretching routine. You don't have to stretch for a long time before your aerobic activity; just a few minutes is fine. I do recommend a three to five minute warm up period before any stretching. This warm up period could be jumping jacks, or running in place. As you will see, stretching can be the source of many an injury. Should you stretch anyway? Absolutely, but safely.

Working out in "stints"

What is a stint? Stints are relatively short periods of time. I call a workout stint any activity that is continuous for about 15 to 20 minutes. As you get older, it's much easier on the body in general to workout in stints. It's also easier on the mind and alleviates the stress of working out. This is what I personally use for my daily exercise routine. I might do one stint on one day and six stints the next day depending on the amount of free time I have. Remember, workout stints can be any activity that is continuous, so that means walking the dog, rollerblading, jogging, yoga, pilates, any activity you can think of. If walking the dog takes 40 minutes, that is two stints. It's easy to count how many stints you perform in one day. I personally like working out in periods of about 20 minutes because I don't feel bored and it lets me have a varied workout regime. I often do 15 to 20 minutes of aerobic activity then follow this by 20 minutes of weight lifting.

Weight lifting

Weight lifting is a very popular form of exercise, especially since Arnold has become governor of California! It can be fun to "build" your physique. It's also great for building tonus in the whole body. The areas you have to be careful of when weight lifting in the gym, are when using free weights. Lifting the free weights off of a rack and moving to your bench to perform the exercise is usually where injuries occur in gyms. Using weight "machines" are usually fairly safe and these machines are usually ergonomically built to not injure the spine. Just be careful when exercising, especially with weight, that you don't flex the lower back while doing the exercise. There are many great home exercise equipment pieces available that will give you resistance to build your muscles without injuring your spine. Some companies like Total Gym sell fantastic pieces of equipment that use your own body weight as resistance to build you muscles. Another great home gym piece is the Bowflex which uses plastic bars for weight resistance. Take a look for yourself, many are worth the expense with gas prices going higher!

Note: Weight lifting as you get older is a great thing to do. As you get older, usually your muscle mass goes down and your overall fat increases. Weight lifting combats this. Doing resistance exercises builds your muscle mass and increases your blood flow. Having more muscle mass makes your metabolism higher meaning you will naturally burn more calories during the day and night! This process of weight lifting will not only make you stronger and look better but it can actually keep you leaner! Start out slow at first and work up to a 20 to 40 minute weight lifting regime.

Chapter Six

....

Kiso Stretching

As we get older, stretching becomes more essential to maintaining health. When I say the word stretching, I also include yoga in this category. You must stabilize your low back before stretching. You may have the idea that I don't like stretching. Actually I've been a proponent of yoga for more than 30 years. I not only see yoga as a one-stop shop for stretching techniques, but also as a spiritual and relaxation tool as well. For many, yoga is a whole way of life, and, no wonder, yoga means union with God. Yoga actually, in its truest form, encompasses every aspect of life from birth to death. So most all traditional stretches are found in yoga, and many non-traditional stretches as well. But the biggest advantage of doing yoga as opposed to another type of stretching regime is that yoga integrates one's breathing, which is a fundamental but often forgotten necessity.

Things to keep in mind before performing Kiso stretching

1. When stretching put an emphasis on keeping the lordodic curve in the neck and low back regions of the spine. You can slightly move into flexion, but be cautious.

2. Doing the slight physically imperceptive oscillation during the maximum stretching portion of some of these stretches will allow you to become more flexible. By oscillations, I mean once you stretch to your maximum, (which means when you feel you have reached your maximum stretch with very slight pain. In other words, if you stretched a bit more you would feel pain). Once in this "maximum" position, you back off slightly for a half second and go forward again stretching to maximum again. This half second back and forth movement is the oscillation I'm talking about. It's done quickly, about one oscillation per half second. You don't have to do this in all stretches but only in those stretches that you feel overly tight in.

3. Finally, the breathing method: During one stretch, a person goes through three cycles of breathing. The cycle varies from person to person. So when having a stretch class, for example, all participants will go at their own pace. This is a necessity. Trying to "keep up" with the rest of the class, starting and ending at exactly the same time is not a good thing because if you don't go at your own pace, you will not be able to get the most out of the session. The breathing cycle will vary with physical conditioning and age. The cycle is simple but profound. Breathing in (inhalation) takes approximately 4 to 10 seconds, while breathing out (exhalation) takes about 12 to 30 seconds. In other words exhalation should take about three times longer than inhalation. I find this time frame fantastic for the integration of the spiritual with the physical while stretching.

4. Also breathing through the nose helps turn on the para-sympathetic nervous system and will greatly relax you compared with breathing through the mouth. This goes back to the flight or fight defense mechanism. When your scared, you immediately open your mouth to gain more oxygen. So when you stretch with your mouth open it increases the sympathetic nervous system. It's all connected!

After a stretching routine, you should feel a powerful parasympathetic rush. The parasympathetic nervous system is the restorative part of the nervous system. If you recall, there are two parts, the Yin and Yang, to your nervous system. We run on the sympathetic nervous system most of the time. It is the "get up and go" and "I'm late for work" kind of response; it makes the heart race and pumps adrenaline to your body for emergency or stressful situations. The parasympathetic part of the nervous system, on the other hand, allows you to take a deep breath and relax.

It is important to integrate both parts in daily life, but the tragic truth is that our modern daily lives are oft times filled with fear and anxiety. Like I mentioned at the beginning of this book, our bodies and minds for the past 160,000 years have been dedicated to living around the campfire, hunting and gathering food, and helping each other. Archeologists believe early homo-sapiens spent hours each day touching and grooming each other (of course we had lice!). Nowadays, especially the older generation doesn't get any touching contact from one another. This is sad – and one of the reasons why I recommend massage to all my patients!

Use Kiso Stretching three or four times a week. It will be a nice addition to your weekly schedule. Before we begin, though, you must categorize yourself. Stretching will fall into three categories. These categories are different than the categories for exercise. This is due to the fact that stretching can injure the back easier that exercise can. The three levels are Level 1, level 2 and level 3. Level 1 stretches are for those who have either no pain or have pain that ranges from a 0 to 2 (on a pain scale from 0 to 10, 10 being the worst). For those on a pain scale from 3 to 5, you should do only level 2 stretches, and for those who are at a pain level of a 6 or 7, you should only do level III stretches. If you are an 8 or above, you should not do any stretching at all because it will hinder your progress towards getting better. Remember, as discussed earlier, stabilizing exercises come first before stretching. You must do at least one week of stabilizing exercises before starting on any stretching regime. We will start with level III stretches and move to level I stretches. Let's begin!

Level III Stretches (pain scale from 6 to 7, moderate pain but not severe)

Wall stretches

Find an area against the wall, lay face up and put your buttocks close to the wall with your legs straight up the wall and feet in a normal relaxed position. Once in this position, your lower back is against the floor. This position supports your lumbar spine and does not allow your lower back to move into flexion while stretching.

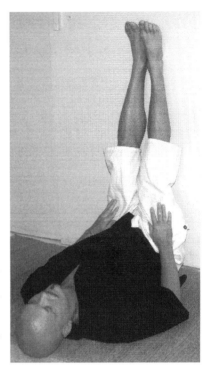

1. First position yourself, buttocks against the wall, legs up.
2. In the second position, allow your legs to go out sideways, stretching the inner thighs. Go as far as possible. Gravity will assist you in this stretch; the weight of your legs will pull your legs apart. You can assist this stretching by using your hands, pushing down on your own inner thighs. Now stretch through three complete breaths as described previously.

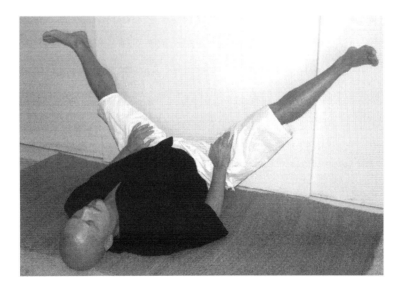

3. Now with legs straight up, hook a towel or a belt over the insteps of your feet and pull back toward yourself, stretching the back of the thighs. Do this three times while breathing.

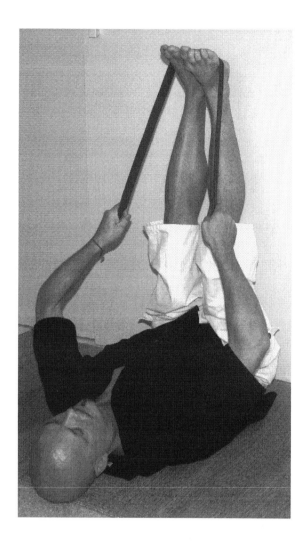

Note: You will notice in doing the wall stretches that it's surprising how stiff your legs feel doing the stretches. This is due to the fact that you are purely stretching your legs. Contrast this with stretching your legs while on the floor, you are "cheating" by using your lower back muscles. It will seem like you are more limber stretching on the floor, but you will be using your lower back muscle flexing the lumbar spine.

Neck Stretches

NECK EXTENSIONS

1. Lay face up on your Kiso Cushion or lay face up on your bed. The Kiso cushion gives you more support which helps push up against your upper back allowing you to stretch the neck further. Beds are quite soft and will not support your upper back

enough to get a really good stretch but it will have to do unless you have a Kiso ball you can put under the upper back where the neck meets the upper back. This will help you get a better stretch while on top of your bed. Another solution is to find a free table top or better yet a massage table in your home. Let your head extend straight back. Allow this stretch to occur. Do this while breathing quietly for about one minute.

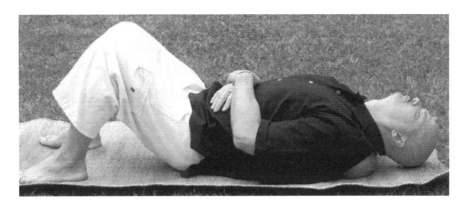

SHOWER STRETCHES

1. Standing in the shower, allow the hot water to beat on the back of the neck for awhile. Once warmed up, allow the head to extend for about 15 seconds. Hold on to something because sometimes when extending the head some folks feel a bit dizzy.

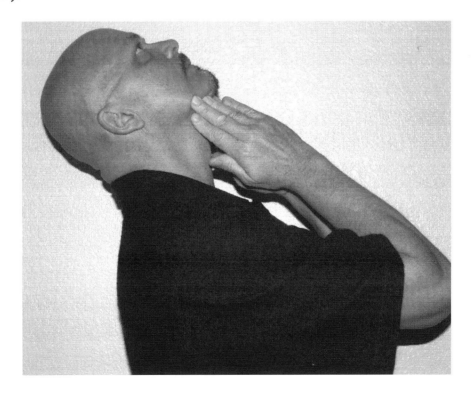

2. Now using your hands push your head over to the side and stretch for 15 seconds. Now do the other side.

3. While standing, look down and with the help of your hands slightly pull down on the head assisting the stretch. Stretch for 15 seconds.

Note; To assist in getting a better stretch, after a 15 second stretch, come back half way from the full stretch and push against your head with your hands for about two seconds and do another stretch. This maneuver will allow you to stretch further the second time.

Gluteal stretches

1. Lying face up on the floor. Stretch your right thigh. Raise the right knee up clasping the right knee holding it close to your body, as close to the chest as you can and do your three breaths.

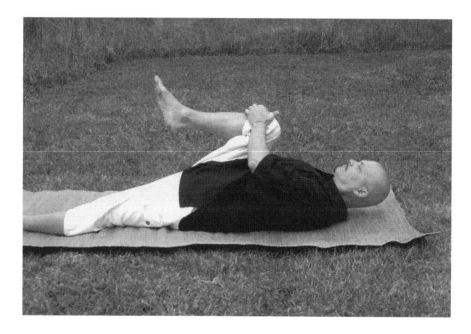

2. Now stretch the left thigh bringing your left knee up clasping the knee in your hands holding it close to your body and breathe. Now do the other knee.

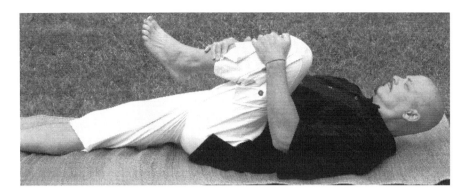

3. Now clasp both knees close to the body and feeling a slight stretch in your lower back.

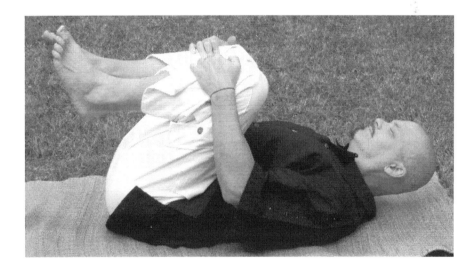

Level II Stretches (pain scale of 03 to 5– moderate pain)

We will start with standing stretches first and end with ground stretches. Perfect them and then commence with a relaxation program.

1. Standing stretch: Stand with legs at shoulder-width apart. Now "activate" your back by sticking out your buttocks slightly and feel the strength in your lumbar spine. This will put a slight lordodic curve into your lumbar spine, which protects it. Now bend your knee slightly (about two inches) and bend forward. Bending forward toward the ground, don't touch the ground. Because you are activating your back,

you will not be able to bend over as much as when you used to bend over and touch the floor without activating your back. The best way to perform this move is to bend the elbows and clasp your hands together. Now bend forward as far as comfortably possible. Do the breathing properly. Inhale, and exhale three times longer. Do this inhaling and exhaling cycle up to three times while in this position. If you feel tight in doing this stretch, try the Kiso oscillation technique to become more flexible quickly.

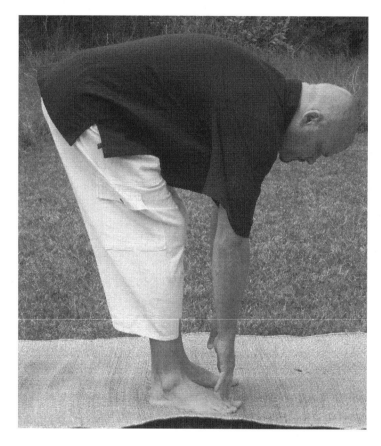

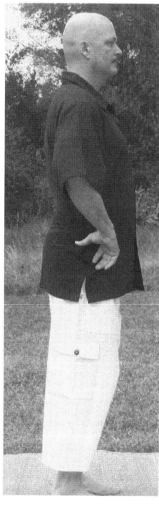

2. Triangle stretch: Stand with legs slightly larger than shoulder width. Let's do the left side first. Point the left foot out left, keeping the right foot in a normal position. Now raise the arms perpendicular to the floor and inhale engaging your back. Now while exhaling raise the right hand up straight above your head and bend over to the left, exhaling while bringing the left arm towards the floor. Finish exhaling. When done exhaling, go back to the beginning position. Now stretch to the right side. You only have to do this once on each side.

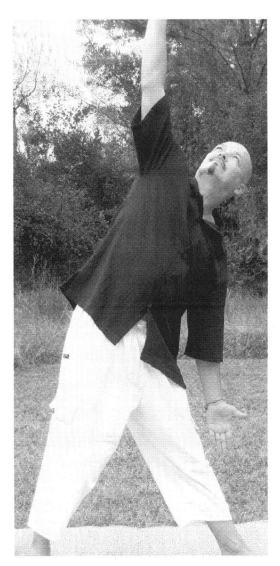

3. Back arches: Stand with feet at shoulder-width apart. Now raise your arms above your head and inhale. Now, while exhaling, arch your low back, reaching above and behind you as you stretch up and back. Do this three times with the proper breathing.

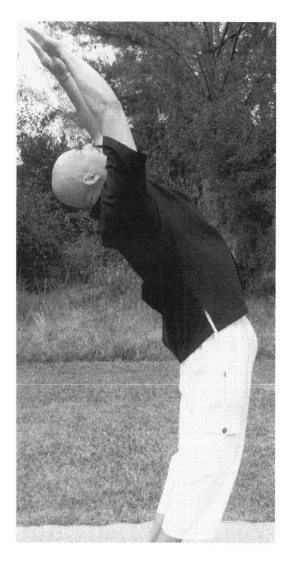

4. Warrior stretch: Again, start by engaging your back with your feet wide apart. Breathe in, now raise your arms above your head, putting your palms together; turn to the left, and exhale, bending your left leg and arching your back and dropping your body down while looking up. It's a great stretch for the low back.

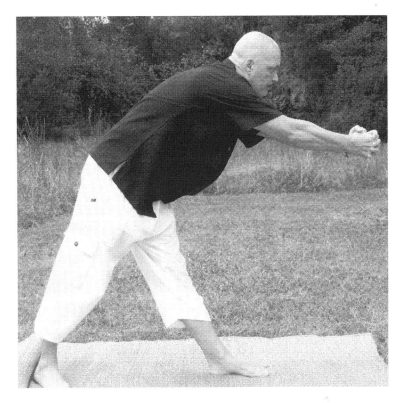

5. Child pose: Sitting on your knees with your feet tucked under you, inhale and then exhale while bending forward bending your upper torso down to the floor and resting your head on the floor, get comfortable with your arms flat on the floor reaching behind you.

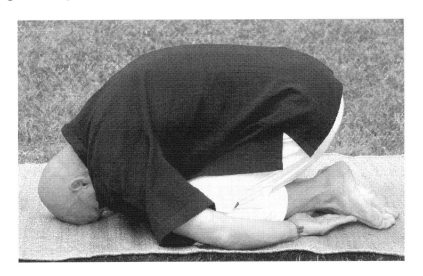

6. Sitting hamstring stretch: While sitting on a chair with both legs bent. With feet flat on the floor, inhale and then exhale and stretch forward while slightly engaging your lower back. Stretch downward feeling the stretch in your lower back and behind your legs. Repeat three times with proper breathing.

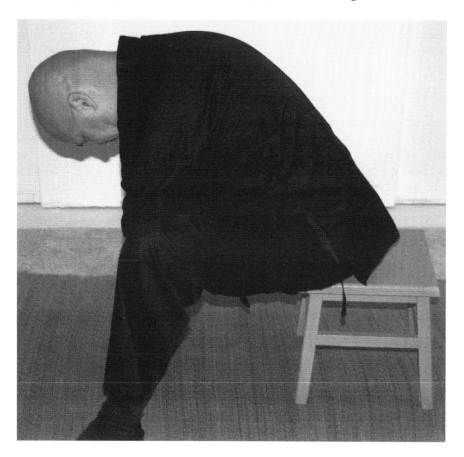

7. Waist stretch: Sit Indian-style and now wrap one leg over the other leg's bent knee. Plant your left foot on the right side of the right thigh. Once in position, breath in. While exhaling, turn your upper torso to the left putting your hand on the ground for support behind your body and the other on the left thigh. Now do the same on the other side. Remember to breath!

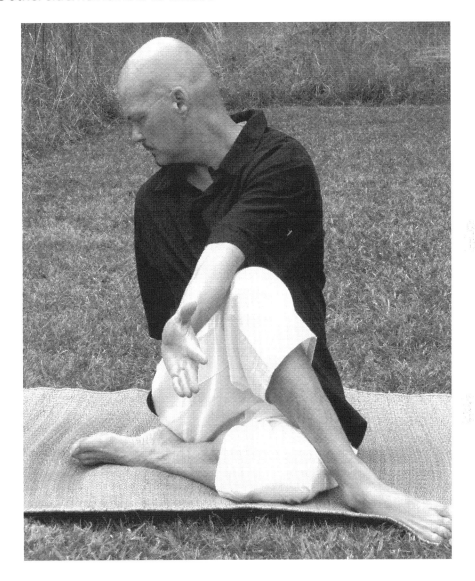

8. Groin stretch: Lean back allowing your upper back to rest on the floor. Keep your heels close to your buttocks. Inhale and now exhale, allowing your knees to rest near the floor both right and left. Now, while still exhaling, slightly push down on both knees to drive them closer to the floor. While in this position, you can do very slight contractions of your thigh muscles going against the pressure exerted by your hands. Now repeat three times.

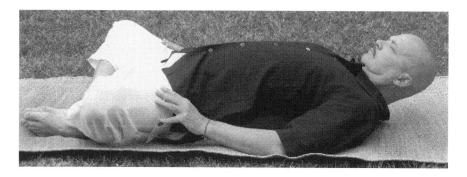

9. Piriformis stretch: (The piriformis is a small muscle that can cause big problems found in the middle of your gluteal muscles). Lying back on the floor with you knees up, put your left foot over your right knee. Inhale. While exhaling, raise your right knee about four inches off the floor. This will put pressure on the left leg and thereby putting pressure on the left piriformis. Now do the other side.

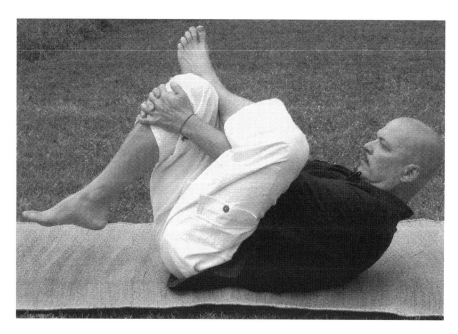

10. Quad stretch: Still lying back, inhale, and turn to the left lying on your side. With the left leg straight, bend the right knee and grab the right ankle and pull it close to you while exhaling. Now do the other side.

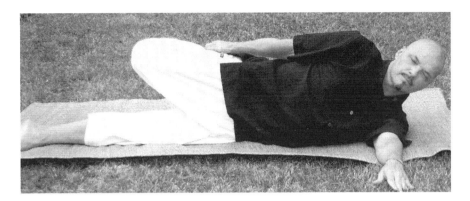

11. Psoas stretch: (The psoas muscle is another muscle found running from the lumbar spine on the inside of your body to the front of the thigh bone, it often hurts when you have a subluxation in the lumbar spine or when your hips are out of balance). Lying face up, first turn to the left and keeping the left leg straight, bend the right knee. With your right hand, grasp the right foot and pull the foot up close to your buttocks and low back creating a stretch in the front of the upper thigh. The more you bring the right knee back the more it will stretch the psoas muscle in the front of the upper thigh. Now do the left side.

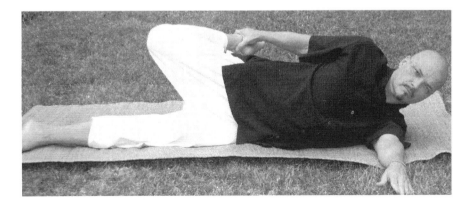

12. Cobra pose: Lying face down, put your hands on the floor as if you were going to do a push up. Keeping your hips and legs flat on the floor, raise your upper torso up off the floor as far as you can without pain. Now look up at the ceiling and do the three breaths. Repeat three times.

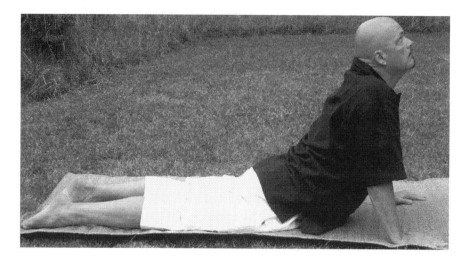

13 . Corpse pose: Lying flat face up, inhale, and totally relax, releasing your hands and feet from their usual positions so that they lie completely loose on the floor. Do three breaths.

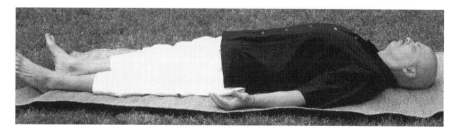

If you had any residual pain after or during this stretching program, note it. If you have a herniated or damaged disc, the slight flexing forward of some of these poses may cause some irritation. Try using the Kiso ball technique to bring relief to the lower back if this has occurred. If you felt neck pain, use the Kiso block or use the meditation cushion to try and bring relief to the neck. Remember, if you have some subluxations, almost any movement can cause a sudden increase in pain.

Level 1 Stretches (pain scale of 0 to 2 - no pain to very slight pain)

You may do all the stretches listed above as well as the following:

1. Forward bending stretches: Sitting on the floor, spread your legs apart and bend forward bringing your chin as close to the floor as you can. Remember to keep your chest straight. Don't round the chest to cheat, doing this can cause too much flexion in the lower and upper back.

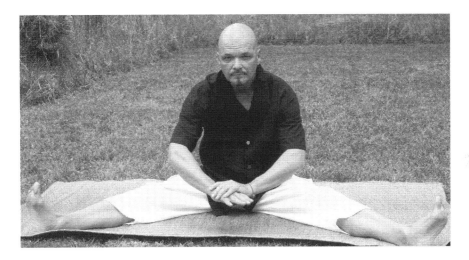

A) Now, in the same position, hold your right leg and use the leg to pull yourself down toward the right knee.

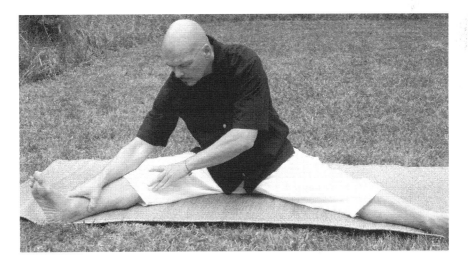

B) Do the same on the left side. Remember to always do your breathing and oscillations.

C) Now put both feet together with legs outstretched in front of you and pull yourself down towards your feet. Remember to breath.

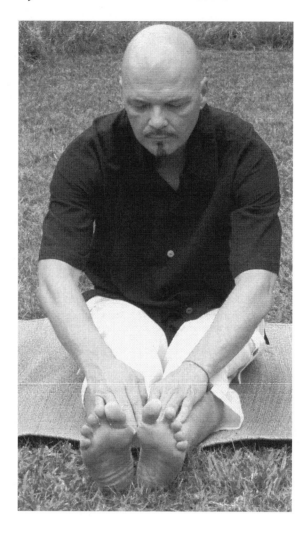

D) Stand and put both feet together and slightly engage your lower back, now bend forward and try and touch your toes.

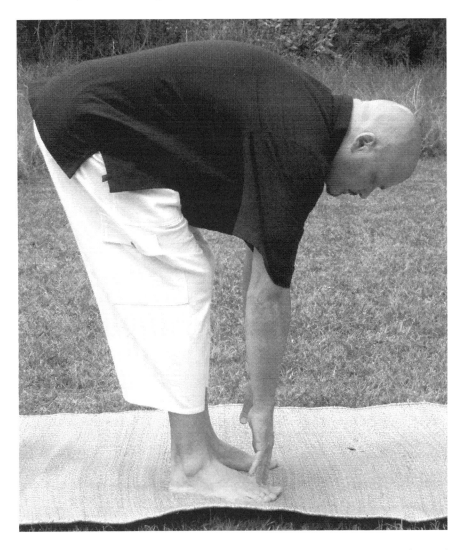

* Why are the forward bending stretches listed together and at the end? It is because these stretches are only to be done by those who do not have any lower back problems, namely, a problem disc. I've seen patients come back from a herniated low back disc and recover and were able to do the above stretches without injury. If you have had a bout of serious low back pain or you are aware that you have a herniated disc, even if you currently have no pain, please be careful when doing the forward bending stretches.

CHAPTER SEVEN

....

De-Stress your life!

Relaxation and de-stressing your life is one of the most important aspects of healing back pain. For some, relaxation needs to be learned. Most of us, in fact, need to learn to relax in some aspect of our lives. We have forgotten how to relax. This chapter on relaxation is very important for back pain. Throughout my 20 years experience I have noticed that when patients have severe back pain, it is usually at a stressful time in their lives. It is usually when they are dealing with big issues, like relationships or moving from one house to another or one area to another. Anything that disrupts the foundation of one's life can always be a source of stress. This stress causes catecholamines, which are released primarily from the adrenal glands, to act like little "pac men" trying to release more energy from the tissues in the body for immediate use to either run or fight. In many cases our stress lasts for many weeks or years at a time. These catecholamines wreak havoc on our bodies and minds. This breakdown of tissues leads to subluxation, which leads to disc injury, which leads to disc degeneration. So it is important to learn how to relax.

About 15 years ago, I had symptoms that I never had before. These symptoms were very strange to me, like muscle twitches all over my body. I also started to have panic attacks. I had never had one before, so I did not know exactly what they were. All of this was manifested because of my innate fight or flight response that we all possess. This fight or flight response occurs when we have stress. The more extreme the stress, the bigger the fight or flight response will be. I realized at this time that I had never really learned how to relax. This goes for a lot of my patients; they go, go, go and don't know when to stop. They don't know how much stress they are putting on themselves. It took me to have a nervous breakdown to realize this. I had two practices and was working six days a week. I had a very active social life, as well as a lot of bills to pay for an extravagant lifestyle. I find this to be true for a lot of my patients. In fact some patients suffering from back pain in their fifties say, "Oh, it's my age, I guess; that's why my back hurts more". I quickly correct them and say that the patients I have that are in the most severe pain are in their 30's. The reason for this is that when you are in your thirties, some have not learned how to curtail certain aspects of their lifestyle. When many are in their 30's, they often drink and party too much. They pile too much stress on themselves in the way of bills and payments, arguments and worry, etc. This leads to perpetual stress, which leads to subluxation. They need to balance their social life with their work life and balance this with an appropriate amount of relaxation and exercise. Many folks in the 20's have a lot of fun, going to college and then start to blend graduating from college to having kids and a family. It's often not an easy time. Also the discs are generally thicker and more full of fluid at this younger age, and because of this, low back pain can be more severe. For those of you who feel that perhaps stress and relaxation along with positive thought cannot help heal back pain, here is some food for thought on the subject. Dr. Emoto has proven that water molecules exhibit different shapes depending on the words that you utter out of your mouth. Amazing, YES! But true. Look at these pictures of water molecules found in lake Baikal.

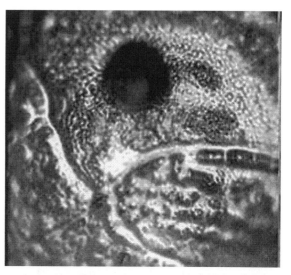

The one on the left was before a ceremony conjuring love and positive thinking. The picture on the left denotes chaos in design while the picture on the right taken after a ceremony of love and positive thought denotes symmetry of design and structure! His work has dazzled communities all over the world. His work is proof that energy from human vibration in the form of thoughts, words, ideas and music affect the molecular structure of water. If, as humans, we are about 70% water, this truth about vibration is significant. There are also numerous experiments proving that cells communicate with each other, even separated by great distances, showing that even tiny cells have consciousness. Deepak Chopra M.D. has written about the evidence that photons have a consciousness and that our brains, bodies and our universe is made up of photons. All this points to the realization that thoughts and vibrations do influence our lives and health. There are thousands of people who claim that reducing stress and learning to relax has made them regain their health and sanity.

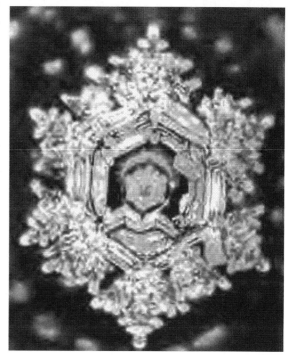

Our innate intelligence is something we are born with. When we skin our knee, for example, we can almost see with the naked eye the healing that starts to take place immediately. Our bodies are made to heal themselves. But with too much stress, the innate intelligence we possess cannot function the way it's supposed to; because of this, we develop illness or disease. While reducing stress, learning to relax and eating well, we help our innate intelligence help ourselves.

Let's get started!
Preliminary Activities to Enhance the Relaxation Exercises

*Prior to doing relaxation exercises, some things you can do to enhance the effects of the exercises are the following:

1. Aerobic exercise during the day or prior to the relaxation exercises
2. Take a hot bath for 20 minutes
3. Practice yoga first
4. Avoid overindulgence of caffeinated drinks

You must find time daily to relax. You should find a clean quiet space in your home where you will not be disturbed for a while. Many people like to light candles, burn incense, play soft music – whatever helps you get in the mood of relaxation is fine.

Relaxation Exercises

Let's start with the easiest and most profound way to learn how to relax. This first relaxation exercise is called the Para-Stim. In this exercise we will stimulate the parasympathetic nervous system. The parasympathetic nervous system makes you relax and to rejuvenate, as I have already discussed. The sympathetic nervous system, which you now know, is the fight or flight part of your nervous system, which makes you sweat, your heart race, feel nervous and worried, etc. It is the Yang part of your nervous system. When it is stimulated, it makes you have anxiety because it expects something to harm you. The parasympathetic part of your nervous system, the Yin part of your nervous system, needs to be in balance with the sympathetic nervous system, to enable you to do many things in your life. For example, to sleep we have to have an active parasympathetic. For sex, we also need a proper combination of the two opposing forces.

Exercise I

PARA-STIM
PHASE 1
Let's start by lying face up. Put a towel, rolled about 3 inches in diameter, under your mid neck and put another towel, rolled up similarly, under the lumbar area about 3 inches above the tops of your hips where the low back has the biggest curve. Pressure in these areas, caused by these towels, increases the parasympathetic nervous system.

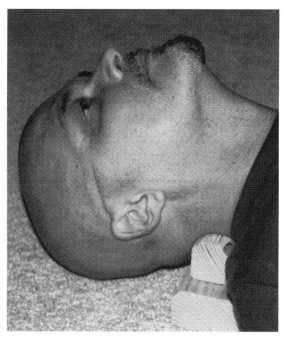

Perhaps you can light some candles and play some soft, ambient music. This exercise" (if only working out was so pleasant!) will take between 45 minutes and one hour the first time. What we are trying to accomplish with this exercise is to get into a parasympathetic mode towards the end of this exercise. You may not feel this parasympathetic state on the first night or on the second night. Those who have been in an extreme amount of stress may not be able to get into this parasympathetic state for one week, but be patient, it will come. The time it takes to get into this parasympathetic mode will decrease the more you perform this exercise. In a relatively short amount of time, you will be able to drop into the desired state in about 5 minutes. Remember to breathe from your abdomen. Breathing from your abdomen also increases the parasympathetic nervous system. You lie there and breathe slowly in and out without laboring. In our American society, we tend to breath from our upper chests. This comes about by having perpetual stress and being in a fight or flight mode. This upper chest breathing may also be due to men trying to look macho or sucking in their stomachs to look better. We are going to breathe in and out for about 5 minutes to decompress from the day's activities.

Phase 2

The second part of this exercise while lying there, is tensing and relaxing all the muscles of your entire body. Starting with the feet, tense the muscles at the soles of your feet for about two seconds, holding your breath slightly. Now release your breath, relax the feet. Do the opposite side of the target area, the tops of your feet. Now tense and release the calf or lower legs in the back and then the front, followed by the thighs, back and then front. Now move on to the buttocks, the waist area, always doing the back then front. Next tense and relax the muscles of the stomach, after which will be the chest, shoulders, upper and lower arms (individually), and then the hands (clench them into fists, release them, and breathe out). Now move to the throat and neck area, then the back of the skull where it meets the neck. Now do the same for the face by scrunching up all your facial muscles, holding as usual the breath slightly and then relaxing the face and letting go. Now at last try to imagine tensing the top of the head and then relaxing. This whole tensing and relaxing should take between 4 and 8 minutes.

PHASE 3

After we have done our tensing and releasing of all the muscles, we will begin the next and final phase. Just lie there and breathe slowly in and out. Thoughts will arise. Don't judge them, but just let them go. If this is the first time you have ever done anything like this, probably many thoughts will come into your mind. These thoughts will slow down the more you do this exercise. Don't get angry with yourself for thinking these thoughts. Just recognize them and release them. Maybe it would help if you imagined them flowing past you like water. Because we don't allow ourselves time to get into a parasympathetic state, we never give ourselves time to cleanse our mind. Have you ever noticed that if you have been extremely busy for a few days and finally sit down to relax, sometimes all kinds of thoughts come into your mind? These thoughts sometimes come to the surface in order to be released. Maybe these thoughts are of anxiety or desires or hopeful expectations of the future or regrets of the past. We usually don't give ourselves time to clear these out, so they remain up in our minds.

You might be wondering, "What if I go to sleep?" Please do not sleep. Actually there is a stage between rest and sleep that you need to dwell in. It is called the hypnogogic state. This state is reached when you get that feeling of euphoria, which is the parasympathetic state that we are after. Falling asleep keeps that from happening. This hypnogogic state is profound and powerful. It is very good for the psyche and very good for your body as well. You may set a timer or just glance at a clock to make sure you have reached your required amount of time for this session. By the way, there are many wonderful alarm clocks that chime with the sound of a temple bell. This is important because the parasympathetic state feels slightly euphoric and once in this state, you don't want to be woken up with a loud alarm that will startle you.

Now, to reiterate what this parasympathetic state feels like, it feels somewhat numbing with a possible tingly feeling all over. You may feel a nice heaviness in the head. Whatever it feels like exactly to you, it will be a truly wonderful sensation. I believe that in this state you receive spiritual energy and that it is also good for creativity and will help you to be in a more positive state the next day.

Note: After a few sessions of tensing and releasing and you feel like you have learned to let the muscles go, you can omit this part of the exercise and just lay face up and relax. Doing the tensing and releasing is to teach you how to let go of your muscle tension. Once you have done this a few times, you will get the feeling of how to release muscle tension in your body.

Exercise 11

SITTING MEDITATION

The next relaxation exercise is the concentration meditation technique. It requires you to sit. Throughout the world all authorities on meditation suggest that you sit with the spine straight. These different authorities on meditation say that the spine, or what is called in the Indian traditions the shushumna, has to be perpendicular to the earth's floor. These authorities say the spine is the spiritual center and must be held in an upright fashion for meditation to be really effective.

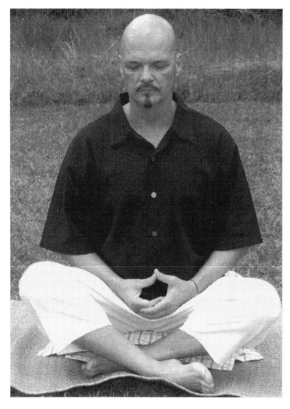

Because you must keep the lordodic curve while meditating you must sit on something that is not only soft enough to withstand 15 plus minutes of meditation, but also makes the lower back straight or slightly curved in a lordodic position. A meditation bench is a fantastic device that not only allows the perfect posture for meditation but it is also soft to sit on and allows the legs to feel more relaxed, so that longer meditations are possible. We sell the Kiso meditation bench on our website, kisolifesystems.com. For people who like to sit on cushions, you must find a cushion (also sold on our web site) that sits you high enough to allow the torso to lean forward slightly, maintaining the lordodic curve in your low back. At first using a cushion may cause you to feel some leg strain, but that should only be until you get used to meditating. In our western culture we sit in chairs everyday. Day after day of this causes the leg muscle to become shortened. In Asian cultures, they squat quite often and sit directly on the floor. All of this lends itself to be able to sit in meditation longer without pain. I recommend that those who have had knee injuries and for those who just cannot "sit" in meditation to sit on a wooden chair. Sitting on a chair is fine because the main reason for this meditation exercise is to learn to relax. A reason for the wooden chair, as opposed to a metal chair, is that wood insulates the energies from the earth and the environment while metal conducts these energies to you. The same conduction happens while sleeping in metal bed frames. Many who meditate sit on the ground with a wool blanket under them to insulate them from these energies. This may seem strange to those of you who are new to this, but I assure you that these precautions are helpful. When you are meditating for relaxation, you don't want to conduct the energies around you. You want to be insulated from them.

When sitting, as I mentioned above, you want to accentuate the lordodic curve. You will also feel like you are leaning your torso forward while your buttocks is planted on the cushion or bench. But what you are really doing is lining up the spine. You are lining up the sacrum with the top of the head. This is why I teach meditation with back care. If you get used to sitting in meditation for longer and longer times, that means that you will have learned to "line up" the spine correctly. That means if you drop a plumb bob from the center of the ear, it will drop through the sacrum in a perfectly vertical line. This is a line of power, and that's why you can see indigenous peoples around the world carrying very heavy objects on their head. It's not because they're "supermen or superwomen"; it's because they have learned to line up the spine, or as I call it the "line of power". If you watch a power lifter, they will get that line of power and actually accentuate it some before lifting. If they did not get this line of power they could be risking the occurrence of a disc injury. Remember when disc injuries occur, it is due to some type of flexion of the lumbar spine.

Sitting Indian style on a cushion is fine for meditation, but if you are more flexible you can sit in the half lotus, which requires you to put one foot over the opposite thigh, or the full lotus, which requires you to put both feet on the opposite thighs. This often takes practice and legs that are very limber and stretched. Another way to sit is to sit with your heels together and knees out as far as possible. Always, while sitting in one of these styles, you should sit with the knees out and as close to the floor as possible. The reason for this is that it stabilizes the sitting posture. Using the Kiso meditation bench is different. Your knees are together and you sit on your haunches. It's a traditional Japanese way to sit called seiza. The only problem with sitting like this is the pressure on the knees. But using the Kiso meditation bench lifts your buttocks up off the floor allowing space between your buttocks

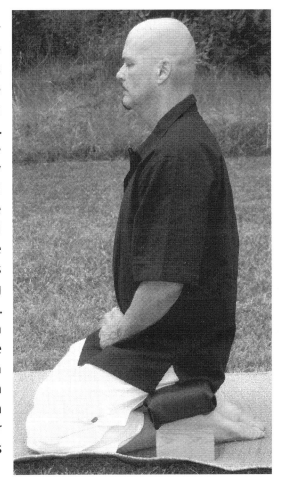

and your legs. It also naturally puts your back into a perfect lordodic curve, a perfect line of power. In a short time you can be sitting for 30 minutes without strain. After all meditation should be about meditation not how well you can do a full lotus!

Get a candle and place it on the floor approximately three feet in front of you. The reason for having a candle flame to look at is that this gives something for your mind to occupy itself with. Sit on your chair, bench or cushion. Get your line of power. The lights should be very dim or shut off in the room, this will allow the candle glow to illuminate the room. Start with a 15-minute time frame. This may not seem like a lot of time, but it may not be easy at first. If you have any subluxations in your spine, these may begin to hurt while doing this meditation. If this occurs, you need to be adjusted by your Kiso Practitioner or chiropractor first. Now, enough said, let's begin.

Sitting quietly, look at the candle flame in front of you. You will be looking slightly down with your eyes but keep your head in the line of power. Remember, although thoughts will come and go, don't worry about them. It may be more difficult than you anticipate, but it is important that you let all thoughts go without judging or pondering them. Sit and breathe, first from your abdomen and then up to the top of the chest. Then reverse the order on exhalation. You should do the above exercise for about one week to get use to it.

Relaxation III

BREATH MEDITATION

Now this will be the same as the above meditation, except we will concentrate on breathing instead of a candle. We will breathe in the following manner: Inhale from the abdomen and then move up again to the top of the chest. This inhalation should last a total of about 4 to 8 seconds. Now at the top of inhalation, hold the breath for about 2 to 4 seconds, now exhale, starting at the top of the chest, moving down to the abdomen as the breath goes out. Exhale about three times longer than inhalation, or about 12 to 24 seconds. Do this for approximately 15 minutes. You should do this exercise for one to four weeks at least 4 times a week.

Relaxation IV

VISUALIZATION MEDITATION

This advanced meditation technique is very good for the mind and body. It requires imagination. This is actually a very serious form of meditation and for those not ready, please do not feel obligated to try this. I include this meditation because it can be profound. Many people have found this meditation to be the backbone of their lives.

It is a form of kriya yoga. I suggest that if you want to find out more about kriya yoga, go to the self-realization fellowship website for more details.

For this meditation, you will sit as usual and breathe like you did in the last meditation. Inhale for 6 to 10 seconds and hold for 2 to 4 seconds and exhale for 18 to 30 seconds. You will note that the breathing times are slightly longer due to the fact that before doing this meditation, you should have practiced the preceding meditations for approximately one month if not more before commencing on the practice of this meditation. "Blood follows breath." This means that if you slow down your breathing, your pulse and heart rate will slow down also. Begin by sitting. Tense the perineum, which is a muscle located between your anus and your genitalia. Tense this muscle two or three times. Bring your mental energy down to this area. Now visualize the first chakra as the color red, it's in the area of the perineum. (chakras are energy wheels that collect spiritual energy and direct it into the body, there are seven major chakras). Now continue up to the second chakra, located below the navel and visualize it as the color orange. Yellow will be the third charka, it's in the area of the solar plexus. Green the fourth, at the heart. Blue the fifth, located at the throat. Indigo the sixth, this is located between the eyes. And finally the seventh chakra at the crown, will be gold.

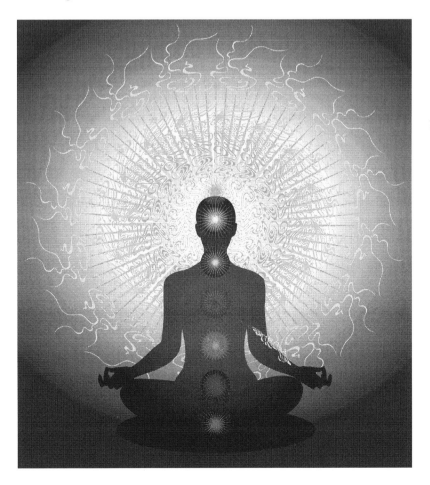

Now hold these energies at the top of inhalation. You might want to say an affirmation here, like "I'm healthy" or whatever you like, while holding your breath for 2 to 4 seconds. Now the entire trip up the spine takes from 6 to 10 seconds. Now for the exhalation. Starting from the crown chakra move down through all the chakras visualizing each of them, going down the spine, one by one until you reach the bottom again. This trip down should take about three times longer that the trip up, so it should take from 18 to 30 seconds. Try this for 15 minutes at first. You can use beads, which we sell on our website, to count the cycles of breaths. Many practitioners do a certain amount of breaths instead of a certain amount of time.

One more thing about relaxation. On the journey to healing myself after getting sick from stress I moved to Hawaii. After moving to Hawaii it was fascinating to watch my own healing process. The fight or flight response was leaving me altogether, but slowly. I attribute this healing not only to the lovely lifestyle in Hawaii but also to the alignment of my atlas and occiput so as to not cause my fight or flight mechanism to be stimulated. Every time I would visit California, I would awaken during the night in the house I grew up in and think, "I feel different!" How did I feel? Why did I feel different? I kept asking myself those questions. All of a sudden the answer came to me.

The "ahh factor"

What is the ahh factor, you ask? For me, it is sitting at home in Hawaii and looking at something beautiful, such as my green yard, for long periods of time. During these times of relaxation, I would sigh "Ahhhhh" while looking at the yard. I believe this was a major factor in my road to recovery. It is very easy in Hawaii to find places with the awe factor. I can simply drive to the ocean and sit on my lawn chair and "drink" in the waves with my eyes, feel the cool breeze, listen to the sounds of birds, and smell the tangy salt air. But, of course, not everybody lives in Hawaii. However, there is beauty everywhere. Even if you live in a city, you can build a meditation room, for example, and put that awe factor in that room. Wherever you are, if you learn how to look for beauty, you will find it and then sighing "Ahhhh!" may come as naturally to you as breathing.

CHAPTER EIGHT

....

Relaxation

Sympathetic override occurs when the sympathetic nervous system runs amok, overwhelming the parasympathetic nervous system. This immediately upsets the digestive system because the blood that circulates in and around the stomach and intestines is shunted from this area in order to be circulated to the arms and legs, for example, if you are running from a bear. Not only does this cause stress, but also creates stomach problems due to this lack of blood flow. The lining of the stomach and intestines are protected by normal blood circulation. During a sympathetic override (such as running from a bear), the stomach lining becomes irritated and ulcers may start to form. All this blood shunting is supposed to help us. It is an inherited defense mechanism from our ancestry. We are supposed to run from the bear and once we escape (supposing we *did* escape, of course), we can relax again. The problem with our society is that the source of this fight or flight response may be the stress of our mortgage payment or an ongoing problem with our spouse. Prolonged stress is what really does the most damage to us.

Other symptoms of Sympathetic override (SO) are the following:

• Not being able to take a deep breath
• Rapid heart rate
• Rapid breathing
• Sweating
• Anxiety for no apparent reason
• Panic attacks
• Dizziness
• Fatigue not helped by caffeine
• Eyes are sensitive to light

These are just some of the symptoms of SO. Basically, in SO, your body is on alert, ready for some type of attack. Our society basically runs on fear. Just look at the basic sample of commercials. They plant suggestions in your head by asking if you have any bad symptoms. You hear these suggestions either consciously or subconsciously, either way, they are planted inside you. You might even say to yourself, "Well, I don't have any of those symptoms yet." Then starts the legal disclaimer asking you, basically, if you don't mind nosebleeds and kidney failure as well as other complications that the product, which they are trying to sell, may give you – lots of bad info, which we don't need! We've got to protect ourselves from all these negative suggestions.

What can we do, you ask? Here are some suggestions.
This area is very personal and I only offer suggestions because all the suggestions below will influence one's lifestyle. Some will find the suggestions absolutely

unsuitable for them, while others may find them helpful. I have categorized all these suggestions into particulars of a person's life.

1) Work

A) Dislike your job? Find a new one you like!

B) Reduce the amount of hours you work. Maybe you can either reduce the amount of hours you work by asking your employer. If you work for yourself, cut your own hours.

C) Cut your commute time. If commuting takes time, try and come to work at a different time or move closer to work, or better yet work at home.

D) Stop trying so hard at work; instead, be more efficient (work smarter, not harder). Don't beat your head against the wall to make more sales. Learn to be content with what you have and not push yourself to make more money. Our society wants us to keep pushing. They want you to be dissatisfied because it keeps you spending money. They don't care if such living is bad for your health. Your well being is worth far more than some quota that must be met set by your superior.

E) Do relaxation at work at least once a day. Find a place to relax daily while at work. If you have a workstation, do relaxation exercises in your chair. You can also just take a nap for a few minutes (preferably at lunchtime, so you don't have to worry about getting caught by your boss, which is another stress you definitely don't need).

Remember, the relaxation exercise 1. At first it takes about 45 minutes to an hour to get into that parasympathetic mode. But with time you can drop into that mode in about 5 minutes – I guarantee it!

F) While at work, THINK POSITIVE! I'm serious. You will have more energy. Don't gossip or talk about negative things. You will be surprised how much energy you will have at the end of the day!

G) Eat well at work. See the diet portion of this book at the next chapter.

2) Home

A) Avoid chaos at home! I cannot stress this enough. I believe in everybody at home using headphones whenever they are listening to the TV, computer, or even music. The sound quality is better and it makes your house peaceful.

B) Play uplifting soft music at home. Light classic and New Age are great choices to play at home. If you have kids, they may start to like it!

C) Do not talk of negative things at home; don't watch stressful shows on television. If you like action movies, use head phones and "decompress" with meditation or reading something that makes you feel good afterwards.

D) Do Yoga, Tai Chi, or some type of stretching regime that allows your stress to be released from the day. Doing this consistently is the key.

E) Do not ever (if possible) use foul language at home. I believe we create much stress and negative emotions with such words and in the spirit that they are spoken in. We attract what we think and say, so don't cuss and use foul language because of the negative "vibrations" they give.

F) Eat well at home. I believe in enjoying life so if you want to have a snack at home do it earlier in the day. Evening snacks are not good for you.

G) If you drink alcohol, drink moderately. Wine and good beers are healthy alcoholic drinks. Brandy is one of the only alcoholic beverages that creates an alkaline-acid base balance in the body, which is a desirable thing. Too much alcohol, however, can interfere with meditation and exercise, even on the day after, so be mindful.

3) Sleep

A) Studies have found that sleeping 6 hours a night is better than sleeping 8 hours. In other words sleeping 6 quality hours per night is about right. Of course some people need less and some more, but I was surprised that less sleep is more beneficial for health and longevity than more sleep. The trick is sleep well and sound. You might try earplugs if noises bother you. Here are some other tips.

B) Avoid coffee or caffeinated drinks. Coffee seems to be the worst for causing stress and panic than other types of caffeine. I know that teas have the same amount of caffeine as coffee, but there truly does seem to be a big difference in the amount of ill effects that coffee causes compared to teas. If you are taking a constitutional homeopathic remedy, coffee is a no-no because of the oils found in coffee. Green tea is a powerful antioxidant and does not seem to cause the adverse effects that coffee causes. Chai is also a good choice. It's been a favorite in India for millennia! Other nice teas to try are mate tea from South America. Of course black teas found in England are great with a touch of milk and two sugars. But if you have trouble sleeping, try cutting out the caffeine!

C) Sleep and awake at the same times everyday. Rhythm is very important. If you get too much sleep one night, the next night it might be hard to sleep well, then the next night after that you will have to "catch up" on sleep again.

D) Sleep on a good mattress. A nice comfortable, but supportive mattress is a help when it comes to having a good nights sleep.

E) Routines are good too. Reading before going to bed helps you mentally get prepared for sleeping. Meditating before bed is also good. Not eating before going to bed is a plus. Also exercising during the day helps get your body tired enough for a good night's sleep.

4) General Lifestyle Guidelines

A) Don't overextend yourself when it comes to extracurricular activities, such as get-togethers and parties. They can be fun but they can also be a stress.

B) Make friends with those who DO NOT bring chaos into your personal life. You will know right away when a "new" friend brings chaos into your life through conversation or constant asking for favors (being "needy") to get them out of situations without really wanting to change the problem that created the situations in the first place. Some people live for chaos!

C) Don't overextend on debt. Try and get rid of credit card debt. Sometimes refinancing the house or a debt consolidation loan can bring credit card and other debts under control. Pay cash for the things in your life, from stereos to cars. I drive an old pick up to work to remind myself that I don't NEED a new expensive car or truck. It also reminds me that if I buy a new Mercedes, I will have to work more! Do I want to work more? NO!

"The Easy Life"

Some people have an easy life. Some are lucky and were given it, while others created it for themselves. How did they create this easy life? By choices, or willful changes made one at a time day by day. If you are not one of those that were "given" the easy life (by inheriting a few million dollars, for example), you are like most of us. You have to make a decision. Do you want stress? Do you want to drive an expensive car, even though you will have to work more every month to pay for it? Not me. Look at the "hippie" way of life for a moment. When we think of the hippie life, we think of not working much and traveling around with a backpack, or driving an old Volkswagen. That's one extreme. There are many variations on this theme. If you don't have much debt or no debt, you pay cash for everything. Because your bills are low, you don't need to work as much or you can work at what you like doing. I know some folks who live the hippie life but have a house or a car paid for. They have done it little by little, and when it comes time to retire, it is a whole lot easier!

Working out and leisure activities

Don't let exercise stress you out. I've seen many patients who are extremely anxious, nervous, and chocked full of stress. Why? because of exercising too much, too long, and too hard. ANYTHING IS A STRESS THAT IS FELT AS A STRESS TO EITHER YOUR MIND OR YOUR BODY! Yes, exercise can be a stress. Even an activity that you consider "fun" is a stress if your mind or your body experiences it as a STRESS! One time I went wind surfing with a new friend. It took two hours to get there by car. Then we unloaded the equipment, waited for wind conditions to improve, only to give up, to reload everything and drive two hours to go back home! NOT FUN! So be careful what you bring into our lives. Keep your plans simple and realistic.

CHAPTER NINE

....

Diet

I don't believe in taking a ton of vitamins. Our bodies are made for surviving and geared for homeostasis, which is our innate ability to repair ourselves and to live in optimum health. As mentioned a few times in this book already, our bodies are made to synthesize substances as food that we have eaten for the past 160,000 or so years. Eating something out of context is like taking a word out of context, which renders it meaningless or misunderstood, at best. If we take a B1 vitamin, for example, 3,500 % over the RDA (RDA is very suspect in itself, I'm only using it as an example), the body does not know what to do with this "out of context" substance. It's a stress on the body. The body only will use a small amount of the nutrient and the rest…well…goes to urine.

Vitamins for your body should be obtained through eating and drinking. Green drinks are particularly rich in vitamins. Most of these drinks contain phyto-chemicals, which are naturally-occurring chemicals from photosynthesis. The sun plays a huge role in making and synthesizing plant growth. These phyto-chemicals are excellent for your health and are in all green drinks to some extent. I believe that taking large doses of vitamins daily is not good for health. Why? They are broken down into smaller particles by our digestive systems, and this in itself can be taxing to the body. Have you ever noticed how your urine turns green after taking vitamins? This is due to the body not absorbing all the particles of the vitamin taken. All these particles and substances have to be synthesized by our organs to be used in our bodies, and especially tax the kidneys. I believe it's one of the major reasons that people have kidney stones (another is ingesting too much salt or calcium). These sources of substances are absorbed into our blood through osmosis, drawing more water into our blood and possibly creating high blood pressure. Our kidneys have to regulate this effect by constantly filtering our blood. In this process, the more substances that have to be filtered out, the more our kidneys have to work. Keep in mind; it is not only our kidneys that have to work to maintain homeostasis but also all the organs of the body working together. Personally, every time I've taken a vitamin, I've felt nauseous. My body was trying to tell me something!

Here is a list of some great greens that may be taken solely or that you may find as ingredients in a green drink:
*wheat grass
*barley grass
*chlorella
*kumat
*alfalfa
*green tea
*spirulina

This is just a small list, but you will find a recommended green drink on my web site. The choice is yours.

Other considerations

Things to consider when taking something green is "the fresher the better"; in other words, deciding which is better, a green drink that has been in powder form and sitting in a warehouse for a year or grinding your own wheat grass, is a no-brainer. The wheat grass would, of course, be a better choice, but for most people it is a lot easier taking the green powdered drink than grinding their own wheat grass everyday. I do believe that taking a powdered green drink is better that taking a vitamin pill, especially one that was not obtained at a health food store. Many of these types of vitamins found in your average grocery store are made with gums that are very hard to digest. I've seen many an undigested vitamin on my patient's x-rays, just sitting in their stomach and intestines.

Other considerations in regards to eating fresh things are vegetables. Cooking and boiling them remove many of the vitamins out of these. Steaming vegetables is much better, or eating your vegetables raw, however, eating raw vegetables in a cold climate can make your body even colder. Getting a juicer is a wonderful way to get natural nutrients into your body. It may sound like I am contradicting myself when I say that in drinking green tea, you should be careful. Yet for some, green tea is a stimulator that can make sleep difficult, causing restlessness. Also, Kelp and Iodine can increase a hyperthyroid condition. Reading the labels of these green drinks is essential, although they are generally good for you.

How about diets? What's good?

Let's modify the word 'diet' a bit. It usually means a short-term way of eating to lose weight. What it really means is a way of eating every day. What is your DIET? Mediterranean? Asian? Or the good old American diet of hot dogs, hamburgers and French fries?

What's the optimum diet?

There has only been one diet that is found to lengthen your life. Only one! The reduced calorie diet is the only diet in the world that has been clinically proven to lengthen your life. In fact it can lengthen your life by as much as 30 percent. There is a thing that occurs in our lives constantly that is called OXIDATION. The more food we eat, the more digestion has to occur, which means that the more oxidation also has to happen. Did you know that the more we eat, the faster our cells die! WOW. It's true. The more you eat, the more your body has to synthesize substances. This causes the cells to die at a faster rate.

Consider your body as a filter. The more you have to filter, the quicker your body gets used up. Or you can look at it in another way. Your body is a lifetime battery. The faster you use up this "lifetime battery", the faster you burn up your life. Constantly digesting food uses up this battery. Another good thing to do is to eat many small meals during the day rather than three big meals. This does not overload your digestive system as much and is more conducive to weight loss. What I'm saying is a true fact, but which is often overlooked. Between meals, you can "snack" on peanuts, raisons, oats etc., and not get so hungry waiting for your lunch or dinner hour.

The best diet by far are plant based diets.

Plant based diets are basically vegetarian diets. It is a known fact that when you are a true vegetarian, you live longer. You are healthier. You get rid of a huge percent of all the world's diseases. If you are a vegan, meaning a vegetarian plus not eating any dairy products at all, you can get rid of up to 70 percent of the known world's diseases. Although being a "vegan" is much more difficult and requires much more expertise in knowing what to eat to get enough protein and nutrients (although our need for protein is much less than most people think). Another hidden benefit of being a vegetarian is that if you eat right, you will decrease your total caloric intake compared with a meat eating diet. This alone can benefit your life and therefore extend your life. It is naturally a reduced calorie diet.

Cancer and a plant based diet

For those who are looking for a "cure" for cancer, don't ask the AMA (American Medical Association) or even the American Cancer Society. They only use "conventional" means to fight cancer. Conventional ways are chemotherapy and radiation along with surgery. Chemotherapy and radiation are dangerous and devastating for your immune system. The outcome of these "therapies" are no more spectacular than a placebo pill (sugar pill). Often times, after going through all of these procedures, the cancer returns. Why? Because they did not address the issue of WHY the cancer came in the first place.

What causes cancer

There is a book that will blow your socks off called the [1]It was written by T. Colin Campbell PhD. This book was written about a study done by Cornell university and Oxford university that studied 65 countries in rural china back in the 1970's and

---

1   The China Study, BenBella Books, Inc. 2005-2009

1980's. The author started out believing that cancer could be cured by protein. As he researched this position, he found the opposite. Injecting rats with a carcinogen (cancer causing substance) all the rats became infected with liver cancer. When He gave the rats a 20% protein diet, 100% of the rats died. When he gave the rats a 5% protein diet, 100% of the rats lived. The more protein he gave the rats, the faster the rats died. From this study, they found that a plant based diet, vegetarian diet low in protein, cured cancer better than any regime of cancer fighting procedures we currently now possess. In the wake of these findings, many cancer curing establishments formed within the United States. These centers focused their attention on using a plant based diet to not only cure cancer but a whole other host of diseases, such as diabetes, gout, arthritis, multiple sclerosis, lupus, just to name a few. For example, these natural centers were curing type 2 diabetes in 5 to 6 days! Amazing, but true. These centers largely moved out of the United states to, near by Mexico, to escape the wrath of the United States Government and the AMA. The Government makes a lot of money "fighting" cancer and there is no money in fighting cancer for the American Medical Association or the American Cancer Society, using natural therapies. The list of cancers cured by these natural centers is massive.

Basically here is the skinny on cancer. We have cancer cells in our bodies everyday. Our immune system kills them immediately. Only 5% of actual cancer comes from carcinogens, the rest comes from diet and a low immune system. That's why many cancers return or move into other areas of the body because the individuals body with the cancer is allowing the cancer to reside in their bodies. These cancer cells that we have in our bodies, that are killed by our immune system, are "seeds". Some of these seeds are planted in our bodies by carcinogens in the environment (about 5%). However, most of these "seeds" are planted by foods that we take into our bodies. That's why natural cancer and wellness centers concentrate on diet first. What is the biggest cancer seeder in foods? Animal protein! It's animal protein that causes the seeds to grow. It's like fertilizer. Animal protein fertilizes the cancer seeds to grow. So if you eliminate or sharply reduce animal protein in your diet, your chances of getting cancer are sharply reduced. Animal protein also is the cause of the other diseases that strike many Americans. Diseases like stroke, diabetes, and heart disease. At these wellness centers, eating a plant based diet without any animal protein, (that means meat of any kind), cures not only heart disease and diabetes but also cures auto immune diseases like rheumatoid arthritis, multiple sclerosis, and lupus. So in my mind, when I think of longevity, and living healthy, being vegetarian is the number one diet. Also in the China Study, they found that the worst animal proteins that fertilized cancer seeds the most were the proteins from milk and dairy! It was casein protein that got the nod for the worst protein you could eat for fertilizing cancer cells to grow. Casein is found in milk from all the animals in the world. "Milk does a body good", the add campaign for the Milk Advisory Board makes it sound like milk is the thing to ingest for a healthy body~ NOT. There is a wonderful landmark book called Diet for a new America, written by John Robbins, son of Baskin Robbins, famous for the ice cream shop Baskin Robbins. John is a vegan and would not take money from his father's fortune because he would not personally drink milk or eat ice-cream. His book talks about vegetarianism as well as the harmfulness of milk. Great book! You can find more information about this book at foodrevolution.org.

More on Vegetarianism

Many say that we are meant to be vegetarian. This could be true, considering most of the world's animals that have grasping hands are vegetarian. There is a great book written by Harvey Diamond called "Fit for Life". I highly recommend it, though it may not be for everybody, but the concepts are very good. Composed of two volumes, the first part will show you how to eat the right food combinations that can literally change your life. He points out that most digestive problems come about by improper food combinations. Is a vegetarian lifestyle the only way to eat well? No. For many who enjoy meat, a vegetarian diet is just not tantalizing enough. But what I've discovered by reading many books and by my own experience on a vegetarian diet is that we actually get enough protein from eating vegetarian. I know it sounds odd from what we've been told, but it's true. Also, the more heavy protein you eat, the less calcium that your bones absorb. Have you noticed that the animals with the largest bones on our planet are all vegetarians?

Other diets

Other good diets are the traditional Japanese diet. Keep in mind, however, that raw fish can have parasites and can also be loaded with pesticides. Large fish eat other smaller fish, absorbing all their toxins and pesticides that may be found in their bodies. But the traditional Japanese diet is good because it is mostly a fish, rice and vegetable diet. Also the Japanese traditionally eat vegetables and fruits that are in season. This is very good for homeostasis. Eating cold foods in a cold climate (for example, eating a green salad with cucumbers in Siberia in winter) would not be recommended. Substituting brown rice is a good idea, because, basically, white rice has very little nutrition. The Mediterranean diet also has cooked fish and lots of rice and veggies as well, which is very good for you and tasty at the same time.

How about fruit? Many believe that, as human beings, our hands are designed to grasp fruit. Look at the shape of a banana or an apple. They are perfect for the human grasp. Also our teeth are very fruitarian in design. Eat a lot of fruit, especially when it's fresh and as organic as possible, but eat it on an empty stomach. So many times we eat fruit after or during a meal, but this creates a sour stomach. If you eat fruit in the morning or in the afternoon by itself without eating at least two hours prior, you will have no ill effects; in fact, fruit is 70% distilled water! This is great for your digestive tract and helps you eliminate well.

If you love meat, eat it sparingly, combining it correctly so you don't develop an upset stomach. Also, try eating chicken and different fouls. Steaks should be eaten only occasionally because even a lean steak is still about 60% fat! Look at it this way, YOU ARE ONE HUGE FILTER! That's right, you take things in, water, salts, food, oils and must process them through your body. Imagine the grease found in one steak caught in a filter. Yes, your body has to filter that steak too and the grease sticks to things like your digestive tract and arteries! Just keep this in mind. I'm not saying you can't ever have a steak but eat food like this sparingly if you must.

If you eat right and take a green drink daily (or at least 5 times per week), you should feel better. Remember to reduce your total caloric intake on a daily basis, which will help you feel that much better. You won't be taxing your body as much. Also taking a green natural drink or juicing instead of overloading yourself with vitamins will alleviate much of the workload on your kidneys and other organs to maintain homeostasis. If you don't like the taste of green drinks and find it easier to take a vitamin, try taking a very good whole food vitamin and mineral supplement. If they are separate, try taking the vitamin in the morning and the mineral supplement in the evening. Taking a vitamin that has basically all the essential nutrients once or twice a day is fine. It's better than taking many individual vitamins that have large amounts of one substance, for example, taking 4,000 times the RDA for Vitamin B1 would not be recommended!

One rule of thumb: Cut down on white foods. White foods like milk, sugar, creams, salt, white bread, and white flour is a good idea. Reducing these foods and substances tend to make the job of maintaining homeostasis easier.

Baseline essentials

One last thing about nutrition. I feel that for your daily vitamins, you should take a good green drink. But for those who would rather take a one a day vitamin take a good natural vitamin that is rather low on potency like children's gummy bears. Remember, don't overload your body with mega doses! Our innate intelligence is designed to work with less not more. You know you are overloading when after taking a vitamin, your urine turns green in color.

JOINT AND JOINT INFLAMMATION

For joint pain you can take glucosamine for those who are not vegetarian and MSM for those who are Vegetarian. glucosamine is often mixed with chondroitin. This is a good combo for joint pain as well as pain from arthritis. There are some good natural anti-inflammatory products out there that reduce the need for the over the counter anti-inflammatory drugs. Taking a supplement with grape seed extract and pine bark extract is good due to the bioflavanoids present in spades in these substances. You can also find bioflavanoids in citrus fruits, vegetables, tea, cocoa and wine. Taking Omega 3 fatty acids are helpful and also reducing your intake of refined sugars and refined carbohydrates as well as foods that increase the allergic reactions in our bodies, like dairy products. Try taking a supplement of essential fatty acids and omega 3. Cooking with olive oil and making salad dressing with olive oil is a good thing to do because olive oil is full of oleic acid a natural anti-inflammatory. Some herbs that are known for their anti-inflammatory properties are:

*Boswellia
*Ginger
*Termuric

SKIN CARE

Some other baseline essentials you may need are skin care products for your body and your face. Using night creams and good organic lotions for your skin is something I highly recommend. By the way, it is now becoming known that sun is not all that bad for you; in fact it's essential. Don't get too much but 20 minutes a day 4 or five times a week is healthy. The sun has healing powers! But too much of a good thing IS NOT a good thing.

HORMONE ENHANCERS

For aging women and men there are some great natural foods and supplements you can take to grow old more gracefully. For women, eating and drinking soy products is helpful for getting a good form of estrogen into the body. Drinking soymilk and eating tofu and miso paste is good for those who are either pre-menopausal or going through menopause.

Men over the age of 40 start to experience a drop in growth hormone and testosterone. Tribulus is a natural herb used for centuries to increase testosterone and testosterone related benefits. It does so naturally. Because it increases testosterone, it increases muscle mass, strength, endurance, muscle and tendon flexibility – and even the sex drive. It also has been shown to lower cholesterol and blood pressure. Wow! Actually rapid heart rate was the only side effect found in certain individuals.

Another "breakthrough" for both aging men and women was the hormone DHEA. It's actually the most concentrated naturally occurring hormone in the human body anyway. But as we age, this hormone decreases every year, up to 90% when you are elderly. DHEA can convert itself into testosterone and estrogen depending on whether you are a man or a women. It converts itself automatically into the right hormone for you. Because it can turns itself into testosterone, it will help build lean muscle and help with sex drive for both men and women. Because this naturally occurring hormone decreases with age, by taking this substance, it's claimed that you will start to feel younger with all the attributes of being young again. I have to caution you that there are basically three types of this hormone found in health food stores, there is DHEA that is synthetic and must be broken down by the liver which puts a strain on the liver and is reported to give you headaches. There is another kind called natural DHEA and another called pharmaceutical grade DHEA. You should only take the pharmaceutical grade DHEA because it has the most desirable effects without some of the other bad side effects.

Because DHEA increases testosterone, it can cause baldness in men. It can also cause facial and unwanted hair in women. It has been reported that it may cause prostate enlargement in men. Other side effects that are worth considering are breast and ovary cancer possibilities not to mention mood changes in both men and women.

Other supplements that have been useful for aging folks are growth hormone stimulators. I prefer the homeopathic kind. These have no side effects and really possess no danger for those using it. I'm very cautious about using supplements and therefore don't recommend using too many supplements and herbs all at the same time. Use them for specific reasons, test them for awhile and decide for yourself if they are working or not.

When using anything homeopathic, remember to not drink coffee with them. It tends to nullify the effects. It's not the caffeine in the coffee. It's the oils found in the coffee. You can substitute coffee with black teas. Black teas are fine to take with homeopathic medicine.

Anything else?

I'm glad you asked. In recent years, longevity has been a hot topic. Many different antioxidants have been shown to help fight cancer and generally keep our minds and bodies from aging quickly as well as keeping us feeling better as we age.

ANTIOXIDANTS

Resveratrol is an antioxidant that is found in red wine as well as the skins of different berries. It is said to not only fight cancer but to also help us loose weight! It also is said to be an antifungal as well as an antibiotic. As with all antioxidants, the active ingredients help to fight free radical damage that not only help cause cancer but that age our bodies. Reveratrol is reported to counteract the effects of estrogen which will boost natural testosterone, which will in effect help build lean muscle mass while decreasing fat stores.

Acai berry is said to be the #1 super food in the world today. It is a berry mostly grown in the Amazonian rain forest. It's a berry about the size of a grape. It's recommended to take about 500mg to 1000mg everyday. It's a powerful antioxidant, so it has all the positive effects that antioxidants provide like promoting the following: higher energy levels, improved digestive function, increased libido, better sleep patterns, anti-inflammatory and younger looking skin just to name a few benefits.

Other great supplements to take that help the brain and memory and help fight the dreaded onset of Alzheimer's disease are the following:

Neuro -PS is a supplement that is used to enhance memory. It has been shown to help those with Alzheimer's disease as well as those who feel their memory has gotten worse for some reason. One of the biggest reasons for a decline of memory is STRESS! This supplement (phosphatidylserine) helps the cell membrane to be more permeable, so cells communicate better in the brain which in turn enhances memory.

Ginko biloba, a powerful antioxident that is well known for enhancing circulation throughout the brain and body. Help mental alertness, enhances mood and generally makes you more energetic. It's totally safe and has been used for years.

CO Q10 (coenzime Q10) helps the heart and cardiovascular system as well as the memory. This powerful antioxidant is also used for it's cancer fighting and cancer prevention properties. It really has no side effects and has been around for a few years now.

CHAPTER TEN

....

The new millennia and the new age of healing

n the past 20 years or so, the subject of healing has taken a new leap forward due to breaking old ties with Newtonian physics. Newtonian physics has been the basis of our science as well as our paradigm for healing sciences for the past several hundred years. Newtonian physics is believable and very predictable both in the understanding of science viewed in it's light as well as predictable in experimental outcomes in the laboratory. Newtonian physics has a direct relationship between cause and effect. However, with the discovery of a new order of physics called Quantum physics, our scientific world has changed as well as our knowledge of healing.

Quantum physics is the study of very small particles like photons and atoms and other particles. The study of Quantum physics has revealed that photons (particles of light) are actually influenced by one another at great distances! Nicolas Gisin, a scientist at Geneva University has led recent experiments on this phenomenon. He is quoted as saying "We don't know how nature manages to produce spooky behavior". Photons that influence each other, thousands of miles apart without any time laps….amazing! Up until now, we thought that the speed of light was the fastest thing around. These photons are reacting to each other thousands of miles apart simultaneously!

A breakthrough film called "What the Bleep do we know" discusses all kinds of interesting topics concerning Quantum physics and healing. One Physicist who was featured in the movie was Dr. Amit Goswami. He was interviewed by Suzie Dagget who asked Dr. Goswami some interesting questions. Dr. Goswami mentions that "Allopathy (conventional medicine) is really emergency medicine designed to keep the physical body alive". He says further that "allopathic medicine and procedures almost always have harmful side effects, they are to be tolerated to keep us alive in an emergency situation". He calls science within consciousness the new science of healing that uses Quantum physics as it's paradigm. While the old paradigm Newtonian physics, cannot answer the many questions that metaphysics imposes, while Quantum physics actually needs metaphysics to help work together to answer questions like the success of homeopathy. Dr. Goswami states "homeopathy--heals without even a single molecule of material part of the medicinal substance". This does not fit with the old paradigm of Newtonian physics but does fit with our new knowledge of Quantum physics.

In the book [2] The Biology of Belief, the author says that an amazing discovery has taken place. That the membrane of a cell is the "brain" of the cell. It's the part that communicates with other cells. This cell communication can happen between cells at a distance. It's all dazzling and fascinating. It's our new world, and it's coming fast!

Let's talk about homeopathy. What is homeopathy? It's an old "science" if you will, that uses the principle that like destroys like. For example, you have watery eyes that

---

2   The Biology of beliefBruce H. Lipton, Ph.D.1st Hay House edition, Sep. 2008

are red and painful. Chopping onions can do the same thing to your eyes. So you take a drop of onion substance and dilute this onion substance with enough H2O or water, to completely overwhelm the original drop of onion substance. This drop of onion "material" is so diluted that it does not exist anymore, or does it. The "energy" from the onion is still present in this homeopathic water. You take a drop of this homeopathic remedy for watery red eyes, (where there is no amount of the original onion "material" left) and you take it under your tongue and immediately your eyes start to get better. Wow, what's happening? We can't explain it with western medicine. Western medicine hides symptoms, it does not get rid of them with something harmless like homeopathy. Yes, homeopathy works and it's been around for hundreds of years, mostly in Europe. It's a wonderful fast acting way towards health that has no equal. A "constitutional" remedy is made for your particular symptomatology. Homeopathy is called vibrational medicine because in it's remedy, there is no original "medicine" left, it's been diluted out by mixing it with water; But the original energy of the substance is still in the remedy and your body can "feel" the vibration. Your body feels the vibration and makes its vibration to counter the homeopathic remedy's vibration taking care of your symptoms naturally. Your health is restored without using symptom covering allopathic medicine. For patients who come into my clinic with "other than physical" symptoms, I prescribe homeopathy to help them regain their health and I've had wonderful success.

In my healing technique called the Kiso Method, there are several phenomenon that have occurred throughout the years that Newtonian physics could not explain. There is an energy pooling that occurs in the area of the skull that can be palpated. It feels spongy when you touch it on yourself or on another person. This sponginess comes about by the cranial-sacral system malfunctioning, causing energy to pool in this area. This malfunction occurs when the 1st cervical and the cranium are misaligned causing the cranial-sacral system to shut down. This in turn can cause anxiety and the fight or flight mechanism to begin. In essence, a sympathetic override happens. The patient will usually, but not always have a headache, can be irritable and will be prone to anxiety. If left for very long (many patients let this go for years on end), the patient can experience all the symptoms of sympathetic nervous system override discussed earlier in this book.

Trigger trauma

One thing I've noticed and have not mentioned in this book so far is that when a person is experiencing a sympathetic override, the patient will exhibit an extreme scoliotic curve. Now, everyone has scoliosis, I've never seen anyone with a completely straight spine. Scoliosis is the bending and twisting a person's spine exhibits. I'm sure you've seen some individuals with an extreme scoliotic curve. One that makes their spine bend noticeably. Many of these individuals have severe pain while others don't have much pain at all. In my manuals I write that you can map a persons scoliosis and determine where a patient's pain will be and how that pain will feel to that individual depending on that person's scoliotic pattern. I tell my patients that you inherit most of your scoliotic curves and those curves that make up that individuals scoliotic pattern won't change much over time. It's their own particular scoliotic pattern, like a finger print, it's unique. But adjusting the spine will "relax" the scoliosis for a while. That's one of the reasons why a patient should come into the clinic and be adjusted about once a month for maintenance. However, having said that, the scoliotic pattern accentuates when a person is in a fight or flight mode. The bends and twists that make up ones scoliosis will be more noticeable and pronounced. Also while the scoliotic pattern is more pronounced, that individual will experience more spinal pain. Now, you ask, what does this mean? Good question. What it means is this, when you come into my office and I detect a malfunction in your cranial sacral system and adjust you for it, you should feel better right away, and let's say you do feel better. Several weeks go by and WHAM! You feel terrible again. Your symptoms came back. But why? This is a common question for patients to ask. "I was feeling so good and all of a sudden the pain returned". Often the cause of this returning pain is emotional. Yes, it's not only possible but frequently is the major cause of spinal pain returning. Remember I said that a misalignment in the upper cervical spine can cause a fight or flight response to happen, which in turn causes a malfunction of the cranial sacral system, well the opposite can occur. A fight or flight moment can happen, either something startles you or you become angry or worried about something and this acts like a "trigger trauma" to the psych. This trigger trauma to the psych awakens the fight or flight response. This fight or flight response causes your natural scoliotic curve to accentuate and WHAM! This accentuated scoliotic curve misaligns the upper cervical spine causing not only physical pain but a sympathetic override to occur again.

In my office I also perform energy healing. I am a Reiki master and have adapted energy healing to compliment my Kiso Method. I use the large nerves in the body to conduct the energy that I pass from one of my hands to my other hand. I can feel this energy and I can evaluate this energy from patient to patient. It not only helps my patients feel better, it also helps them to be adjusted easier. My patients love the energy work and if I forget to do the energy work on them when I'm very busy, they remind me to do it. The energy work I do is called "Kiso Bio Circuitry" and is taught in one of my manuals. The point is, Newtonian physics cannot explain any part of energy healing, how could something unseen influence something else physical or non physical. In Newtonian physics, remember everything is cause and effect, things MUST be seen to really exist. But in Quantum physics, it's excepted that some things don't exist for observation, in fact some things seen can disappear and reappear again right in front of you. In Quantum physics the experimenter can influence the experiment by his or her own intention. WOW! It is amazing, but it's a fact. Quantum physics also excepts the fact that water molecules either have a chaotic pattern or a beautiful pattern depending on what kind of "vibrations" they have received from those around the water. Again, intention, vibration, unseen stuff!

Let's put it in simpler terms. Let's look at ourselves as if we were computers. Our DNA is our hard drive. We have RNA which reads our DNA. The RNA is like a software program that "reads" our DNA. The RNA takes information from our DNA and makes us function. We have many good traits from our ancestry that make us who we are (part of our hard drive again). We may be horrible at math but great at playing guitar. We might have big muscles because our ancestors had big muscles. All of these traits are read by our computer program which incorporates our RNA and is put into motion via our software program. Until recently, we thought our DNA was set in stone. That whatever we inherited from our ancestors we were stuck with. If my ancestors had cancer, maybe I will be prone to cancer. Well, now we know that we CAN change our software program. Maybe originally we had a "negative" software program. We were waiting for things to fall on us like cancer or high blood pressure or diabetes. We knew something bad was going to manifest from our DNA. Through our new knowledge of healing, with the help of Quantum physics as our paradigm, we now know we can change our software program and "read" our DNA in a different way. Instead of inheriting cancer, for example, now we are impervious to cancer. We thrive because our new software program is reading our DNA in a positive way! We no longer have to fear what's lurking in our DNA. Our new positive attitude has made our software program come alive with wonderful new hope and healing that we never thought possible, if fact, now we have a new software program, downloaded and operating!

So when you begin to manifest pain, ask yourself what caused it. What recent possible trauma may have set this off. There is a diagnosis called post traumatic stress disorder or PTSD that can trigger many ailments in the body of those who have experienced it. I believe fibromyalgia is just one of those ailments that has manifested from PTSD. Patients who have had PTSD have to be extra good to themselves and vigilant not to get sucked into negative scenarios that help perpetuate their pain. PTSD can come in many forms. Vietnam vets, Desert Storm vets, children abused by someone and those who have had a nervous breakdown. To an outsider, one may think that another person's trauma was not all that bad. But it's the individuals response to that trauma that makes it a Post Traumatic Stress Disorder. I've had many a patient with PTSD and I know they could manifest a setback more often than most patients. So for them, I make sure they practice some relaxation techniques such as Bio Feedback or meditation. In some cases I encourage them to go to counseling to deal with the PTSD. But through positive thought and less stress, we can change our lives and our program!

CHAPTER ELEVEN

....

Your Personal Healing Workshop

I hope that I have touched upon some valuable information for you. Back pain just doesn't happen because you stepped off a curb wrong or lifted a notebook off a counter. It occurs because of many factors. That's why I have touched upon so many areas in life.

Now that the conclusion of this book draws near, there is one more very important aspect I would like to include now. When in pain, using your mind and imagination is more than helpful in the healing process. It is essential. I will try to show you how to do this.

Find a comfortable area in your home. You'll need about 10 to 15 minutes at a good time of the day or night that allows you to be undisturbed. A good time for this is when you are very calm and in a "good space". In other words, you do not want to do this when you are agitated or when you are in an extreme amount of pain. If your back is in an excessive amount of pain to the point that you find it difficult to breathe, this will definitely hinder the process. Yet even in severe pain there may be times when you have settled down, perhaps you have taken pain medication, or you have positioned yourself to be more relaxed and are not feeling the pain as much. I might add that this process is also beneficial if you are in perfect health and feeling no pain because it will help you to keep feeling better. Lying face up on the floor or sitting in a meditation posture or lying back on a sofa, all are fine. The important thing is to be as relaxed and comfortable as possible. Now, breath in and out, slowly for a few minutes until you are in a very relaxed state. The hypnogogic state is best. Next, focus your imagination on being totally healed. This can be an image of yourself, radiating perfect health. See this image, feel yourself as this image, having no pain, looking radiant and knowing you are in perfect health. Now say to yourself: "I'm in perfect health...I am in perfect health..." Repeat this a few times, and as you do, feel thankful for being in this state of perfect health. Say "Thank You for this state of perfect health." Now enjoy the wonderful feeling of being in perfect health. Feel it! Feel thankful. You are in a very relaxed mode, picturing yourself in perfect radiant health. You are being thankful for the wonderful blessing that has been bestowed upon you.

Now comes the most important part. Relax by lying there and breathing deep and long. No matter what position you are in, get into a "healing point". Healing point is the maximum point of allowing. This is when you "open the door" to allowing this healing to take place. In the healing point, you will feel a kind of numbness, an open feeling of knowing that the healing you desire is now taking place. It is a place where you feel no doubts. It is a relaxed and centered mental space where true healing takes place. Stay in this place for as long as you want to. It can last from 10 seconds to several minutes. Just ride along in the healing point for as long as you can. After your healing workshop, just know that the healing has already taken place. You can use the healing workshop to do all kinds of "healing" in your life, not only healing back pain, but also healing of every kind of "pain" in your life: money problems, stressful areas of your personal life -- you name it! You can bring it into the healing workshop every night if you like.

A brand new day!

My parting words with you: I am sure that you have heard the expression "A brand new day!" Well, it's true! We awaken every morning into a brand new day. I believe in the law of attraction, in other words, we attract into our lives and bodies what's going on in our minds and thoughts. This law of attraction stops every night when we go to sleep. Take advantage of this! Make it a habit to think of pleasant thoughts every night before going to sleep. Think of all the wonderful things that have happened during that day. If it has been a hard day, think about the blessings you have in your life. Make it a point to wake up every morning with renewed appreciation for your life. When waking up in the morning, start by thinking how great the bed feels, how soft the pillow feels against your face. When your feet touch the floor, say "thank you for this beautiful day!" Feel renewed strength and appreciation for having the life you have. Every day IS a new day, make it count, remember to be grateful and that life is a Joy!

Thank you!

*Abraham-Hicks